Clinical

Hyperten

British Library Cataloguing in Publication Data
A catalogue record for this book is available from the British Library

ISBN 1-85315-485-7
ISSN 1473-6845

Phototypeset by Phoenix Photosetting, Chatham, Kent
Printed in Europe by the Alden Group, Oxford

About the author

Gregory YH Lip MD FRCP (Lond Edin Glasg) DFM FESC FACC is Professor of Cardiovascular Medicine and Director of the Haemostasis, Thrombosis and Vascular Biology Unit, University Department of Medicine, City Hospital, Birmingham. His research interests range from clinical (atrial fibrillation, hypertension, heart failure, ethnicity and vascular disease, etc) to the laboratory (thrombogenesis, atherogenesis and vascular biology in cardiovascular disease and stroke). He has published extensively on the clinical epidemiology and pathophysiology of hypertension.

He is a Nucleus member of the European Society of Cardiology's working group on 'Hypertension and the Heart', and is Deputy Editor of the *Journal of Human Hypertension*.

Preface

The management of hypertension has evolved substantially – it is no longer a question of 'should we treat hypertension?' but 'how to treat?' and 'who to treat?' The last decade has seen significant advances in therapy, with well conducted outcome trials and advances in our approach to managing the hypertensive patient.

This book aims to provide a comprehensive overview on hypertension, ranging from the epidemiology and pathophysiology, to clinical features, investigations and management. It is hoped that this book would be of use to all clinicians, nurses and other paramedical staff involved in the care and management of patients with hypertension.

Gregory YH Lip
Birmingham 2002

Acknowledgements

I acknowledge the contribution from my research fellow, Christopher Gibbs, to the chapter on hypertensive 'Urgencies and Emergencies'.

Gareth Beevers painfully endured my discussions and debates, as well as my coloured slide presentations – to him I owe a debt of gratitude for an education in hypertension.

Contents

1. Epidemiology

Blood pressure and cardiovascular risk

Prevalence

Aetiology

Hypertension and the menopause

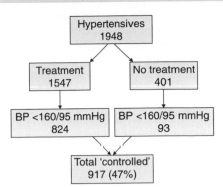

Figure 1.1
Hypertension in general practice in England – illustrating the 'rule of halves'. [Adapted from Poulter *et al. Blood Pressure* 1996; **5**: 209–15.]

> Complications of hypertension include stroke, heart disease, peripheral vascular disease, renal failure and retinopathy

Hypertension is a common problem and a major preventable cardiovascular risk factor. The prevalence of hypertension increases with age. With the increasing age of the general population, the prevalence of hypertension and its complications is likely to continue rising.

Hypertension has few symptoms and many patients will be unaware that they have the condition until complications occur, such as:

- stroke
- heart disease
- peripheral vascular disease
- renal failure
- retinopathy.

The need to treat systemic hypertension is now well established: it is no longer a question of 'do we treat?' but more 'who and how should we treat?'

The detection and treatment of hypertension is vital in the battle to reduce vascular disease – currently the major cause of death in the UK. Despite the advances in antihypertensive drugs, it remains an unfortunate fact that only about 50% of patients with hypertension in primary care are correctly identified, 50% of whom are actually treated and that only 50% of these have adequate blood pressure (BP) control – the 'rule of halves' (Figure 1.1).

Blood pressure and cardiovascular risk

Definition of hypertension

Hypertension can be defined pragmatically as 'that level of BP above which the use of antihypertensive treatment does more good than harm'. This level will vary from patient to patient and balances the risks of untreated hypertension with those of long-term exposure to antihypertensive drugs and their side-effects. This concept of cardiovascular risk has been applied to definitions of BP levels that require treatment.

> Treatment of hypertension requires a balance between the risk of untreated hypertension and long-term exposure to antihypertensive drugs

Almost certainly, patients with a sustained systolic BP ≥160 mmHg or a sustained diastolic BP ≥100 mmHg are clearly 'hypertensive' and should be initiated on antihypertensive treatment. Patients with a sustained systolic BP between 140 and 159 mmHg or sustained diastolic BP between 90 and 99 mmHg are also 'hypertensive' (Table 1.1). The guidelines from the American Joint National Committee on prevention, detection, evaluation, and treatment of high BP (JNC–VI) define hypertension as a systolic BP >140 mmHg and/or a diastolic BP >90 mmHg.

The approach to the treatment of hypertension has changed in that it should no longer be treated as an individual disease, but in the context of a patient's total cardiovascular disease (CVD) risk. Other risk factors need to be taken into account (Figure 1.2), such as:

- diabetes mellitus
- hyperlipidaemia
- smoking
- family history of CVD.

Current recommendations of the British Hypertension Society (1999) advise antihypertensive treatment according to the presence or absence of target organ damage, CVD or a 10-year coronary heart disease (CHD) risk of ≥15% according to the Joint British Societies CHD risk assessment program/risk chart (see inside front cover). Indeed, there is a strong 'additive' effect of other risk factors, such as diabetes, hyperlipidaemia, smoking, gender etc, to the overall risk profile. The charts are based on the Framingham risk function and specifies three levels of 10-year risk: ≥30%, ≥15% and <15%. These three groups are represented by three colour bands on the chart for easy use. The information needed to assess scores is shown in Table 1.2.

In view of the higher cardiovascular risk associated with diabetes, in people with diabetes mellitus, systolic BP that is sustained ≥140 mmHg or diastolic BP sustained ≥90 mmHg requires drug therapy.

Table 1.1 (a)
The definitions and classification of BP levels (WHO/ISH, 1999)

Category	Systolic BP (mmHg)	Diastolic BP (mmHg)
Optimal	<120	<80
Normal	<130	<85
High-Normal	130–139	85–89
Grade 1 Hypertension (mild)	140–159	90–99
Subgroup: borderline	140–149	90–94
Grade 2 Hypertension (moderate)	160–179	100–109
Grade 3 Hypertension (severe)	≥180	≥110
Isolated Systolic Hypertension	≥140	<90
Subgroup: borderline	140–149	<90

[When a patient's SBP and DBP fall into different categories, the higher category should apply]

Table 1.1 (b)
Risk stratification and treatment options [adapted from JNC-VI]

	Blood Pressure (mmHg)	No risk factors, target organ damage/cardio-vascular disease	>1 Risk factor* (not including diabetes); No target organ damage/ cardio-vascular disease	Target organ damage/ cardio-vascular disease** and/or diabetes, ± other risk factors
'High normal'	130–139/85–89	Lifestyle	Lifestyle	Drug therapy
Stage 1	140–159/90–99	Lifestyle	Lifestyle, up to 6 months	Drug therapy
Stage 2 and 3	≥160/≥100	Drug therapy	Drug therapy	Drug therapy

*Major risk factors: smoking, hyperlipidaemia, diabetes mellitus, age >60 years, sex (men and postmenopausal women), family history of early cardiovascular disease (ie women <65 years, men <55 years)
**Target organ damage/cardiovascular disease: heart disease (LVH, ischaemic heart disease, heart failure), cerebrovascular disease, nephropathy, peripheral vascular disease, retinopathy

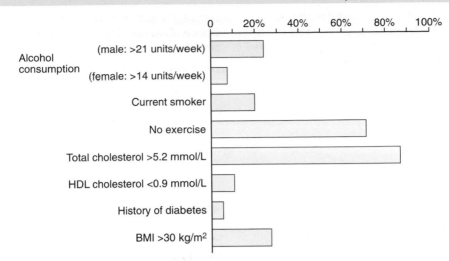

Figure 1.2
Concomitant risk factors in hypertensive patients. HDL, high-density lipoprotein; BMI, body mass index. [Adapted from Poulter et al. *Blood Pressure* 1996; **5**: 209–15.]

Certainly, it is also important to take into account not only the pathological consequences of hypertension but also the psychological and social consequences of labelling a patient as hypertensive, such as difficulties in finding employment and life insurance.

Hypertension and cardiovascular or cerebrovascular risk

There appears to be an almost dose–response relationship between hypertension and the risk of stroke or CHD; conversely, the reduction of BP by antihypertensive treatment reduces the risk of stroke and heart attacks (Figure 1.3).

In 1990, MacMahon et al analysed nine prospective longitudinal observational studies from North America and Europe with large, virtually untreated middle-aged and predominantly (96%) male populations, totalling 4.2 million person-years of observation. After a mean follow-up of 10 years, this meta-analysis confirmed the positive, continuous, independent association of

Table 1.2
Use of the Joint British Societies coronary heart disease risk chart (see inside front cover)

Information needed:	Age
	Sex
	Systolic BP (mmHg)
	Diastolic BP (mmHg)
	Smoking status
	Serum Cholesterol (any units)
	HDL Cholesterol (same units as serum cholesterol)
	Presence of Diabetes
	Presence of LVH on ECG

The 10-year CHD absolute risk (cardiovascular death or non-fatal myocardial infarction) can be found from the charts. In the presence of a positive family history, the 10-year CHD risk should be adjusted by a factor of 1.5 if the patient has a first degree male relative developing CHD or other atherosclerotic disease before the age of 55 or a female first degree relative with a similar history before the age of 65.

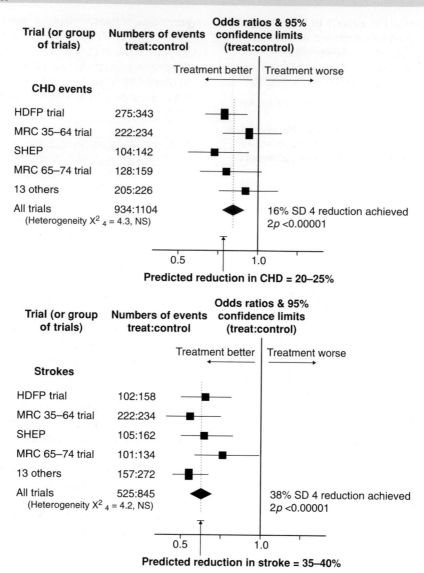

Figure 1.3
The effect of treating hypertension on the risk of suffering from coronary heart disease or stroke. CHD, coronary heart disease.

stroke and coronary risk with high BP throughout its range. The data suggests that a 5–6 mmHg reduction in the average level of diastolic BP would be associated with an approximately 40% reduction in stroke and a 20–25% reduction in CHD. Crucially, there was no evidence of a threshold between 'normal' BP and the pressure associated with higher risk. Furthermore, there was very little evidence in untreated populations of a so-called 'J-Curve', where increased risk might be seen in individuals with low BPs.

> Reducing the average level of diastolic BP by 5–6 mmHg would give a 40% reduction in stroke and a 20–25% reduction in CHD

A lower level of risk appears to be present in women, at least below the age of 55 years. Also, in the Eastern Stroke and CHD Collaborative (1998), a different ratio between heart attacks and strokes is seen among Far Eastern populations.

In the Multiple Risk Factor Intervention Trial, a cross-tabulation of systolic and diastolic BPs found that relative risk of CHD would increase progressively as follows:

- 1.0 with optimal levels of BP (regular systolic BP <120 mmHg, diastolic BP <80 mmHg)
- 3.23 in isolated diastolic hypertension (diastolic BP >100 mmHg, systolic BP <120 mmHg)
- 4.19 in people with isolated systolic hypertension (systolic BP >160 mmHg, diastolic BP <80 mmHg)
- 4.57 in those with a combined increase of both systolic and diastolic BP (systolic BP >160 mmHg, diastolic BP >100 mmHg).

This is illustrated in Figure 1.4. The corresponding rise of stroke risk is also shown.

There has been some debate on the relative importance of systolic and diastolic blood pressure, but in practice systolic blood pressure should be regarded as the more important. In epidemiological studies both systolic and diastolic blood pressure are important risk factors for cardiovascular disease. Certainly, systolic blood pressure is a better predictor of cardiovascular mortality and morbidity, even when correcting for underlying diastolic blood pressure. There is a greater effect of systolic blood pressure compared to diastolic on relative risk of CHD.

Prevalence

The prevalence of hypertension varies depending on the definition used. Using a fairly strict definition of a systolic BP >140 mmHg or a diastolic BP >90 mmHg or current treatment with antihypertensive medication, the prevalence of hypertension varies from 4% in 18–29 year olds to 65% in the over 80s in the US population. Recent data published from the Birmingham Factory Screen project are illustrated in Figure 1.5. This shows the rise in blood pressure with age, as well as ethnic differences.

Nevertheless, hypertension is not distributed evenly in the community, and even in the UK there are variations with geography. For example, in a survey of 24 large towns, the lowest mean BP was found in Shrewsbury, while the highest was in Dunfermline where the BP (systolic/diastolic) was on average 17/11 mmHg higher.

Systolic blood pressure also rises steadily with increasing age and the prevalence of hypertension, including isolated systolic hypertension (ISH), is more than 50% in those aged over 60 years. Isolated systolic hypertension is defined as a BP ≥160/90 mmHg. In fact ISH is the predominant form of hypertension found in this population (Figure 1.6).

On a wider scale differences in BP are even greater, and in some primitive communities, hypertension is virtually unknown. Indeed, studies of migrant populations demonstrate a shift in mean population BP to higher levels in urban dwellers, compared to the rural setting. The reasons for this difference are probably multiple and include differences in diet (including salt intake), the stress of urban living and lifestyle differences.

Many patients with 'high normal' blood pressure levels will progress to overt hypertension. In the Framingham Heart study, 9845 non hypertensive patients were followed-up for 4 years, and their blood pressures were initially classified as: optimum (SBP<120 & DBP<80 mmHg), normal (SBP 120-9 or DBP 80-4 mmHg) or high-normal (SBP 130-9 or DBP 85-9 mmHg). The proportions progressing to >140/90 are illustrated in Table 1.3. These findings support recommendations for monitoring individuals with high normal BP once a year, and

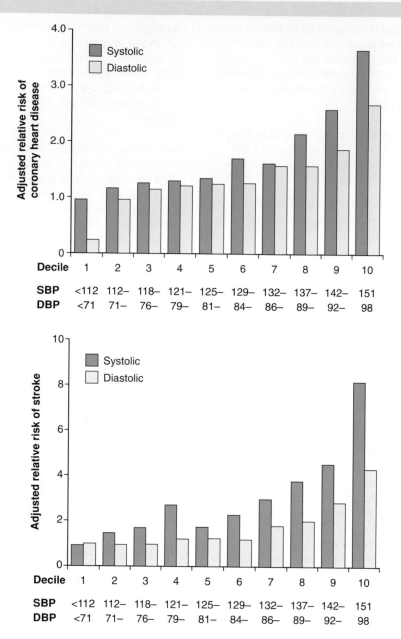

Figure 1.4
How increasing systolic and diastolic blood pressures affect the relative risk of coronary heart disease and stroke. SBP, systolic blood pressure; DBP, diastolic blood pressure [Adapted from Stamler *et al. Arch Int Med* 1993; **153**: 598–615; He *et al. J Hypertens* 1999; **17**: 7–13.]

monitoring those with normal blood pressure every 2 years, and they emphasise the importance of weight control as a measure for primary prevention of hypertension.

In understanding the problem of hypertension it is important to grasp the whole population perspective. In a population, BP is a continuous variable, distributed in a roughly normal (or

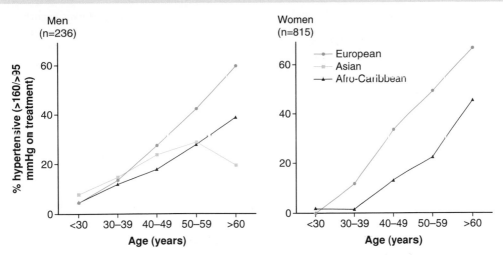

Figure 1.5
How age, gender and ethnicity affect hypertension. [Adapted from Lane et al. J Hum Hypertens 2002; **16**: 267–73.]

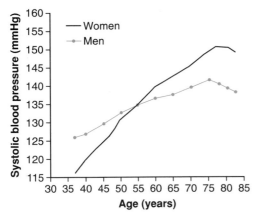

Figure 1.6
Cross sectional age trend of isolated systolic hypertension in men and women. [Adapted from Kannel WB. Am Heart J 1999, 130. 1205.]

Table 1.3
Progression to hypertension in the Framingham Heart Study

	Baseline BP (mmHg)	% progressing to >140/90 mmHg over 4 years
Age 35–64	<120 & <80	5.1%
	120–9 or 80–4	18.1%
	130–9 or 85–9	39.4%
Age 65–94	<120 & <80	18.5%
	120–9 or 80–4	29.2%
	130–9 or 85–9	52.5%

[Adapted from: Vasan et al. Lancet 2001; **358**: 1682–6]

Gaussian) manner. There are not two separate groups of individuals (that is, those with and without hypertension) but a continuous range of BP from the lowest to the highest with the majority of individuals falling somewhere in the middle. Although those with very high blood pressures are individually at very high risk of stroke and CHD, there are relatively few of them, so treating all of them for hypertension would have little impact on the number of strokes and heart attacks occurring in the

population as a whole. Furthermore, most strokes and heart attacks occur in those with only mildly elevated or even normal BP.

> BP is a continuous variable with a normal distribution. There are not two groups – with and without hypertension – but a continuous range of BPs with most people falling somewhere in the middle

The 'population approach' to managing hypertension suggests that reducing the mean BP of the population as a whole by only a few mmHg using public health measures (such as reducing salt intake, increasing exercise etc) would significantly cut the rate of stroke and CHD when compared to the 'high-risk strategy' of achieving large reductions in BP in only a few 'high-risk' individuals.

Aetiology

The vast majority (>95%) of patients with hypertension have primary or essential (idiopathic) hypertension, where there is no immediate underlying cause (Figure 1.7). This definition is somewhat misleading in that all hypertension clearly has a cause, albeit due to the interplay of complex genetic and environmental factors.

Even in so-called 'essential hypertension', there are many influences that cause a raised BP, such as:

- salt intake
- potassium intake
- alcohol
- dietary factors
- exercise
- gender
- ethnic origin
- body mass index.

Acute stress can cause a rise in BP, but there is little evidence of a causal effect of chronic

stress on BP. The so-called 'Barker hypothesis' suggests that fetal influences, particularly birth weight, may be a determinant of adult BP. For example, small babies are more likely to have high BP as adolescents and to be hypertensive as adults.

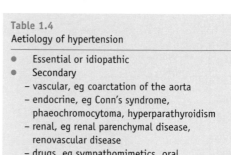

Fetal influences, particularly birth weight, could be a determinant of adult BP

In a small minority of patients, hypertension is 'secondary' or due to an underlying disease usually involving the kidneys or endocrine system (Table 1.4). Effective treatment of the underlying condition can sometimes abolish the hypertension.

Table 1.4
Aetiology of hypertension

- Essential or idiopathic
- Secondary
  - vascular, eg coarctation of the aorta
  - endocrine, eg Conn's syndrome, phaeochromocytoma, hyperparathyroidism
  - renal, eg renal parenchymal disease, renovascular disease
  - drugs, eg sympathomimetics, oral contraceptives
  - pregnancy
  - genetic syndromes

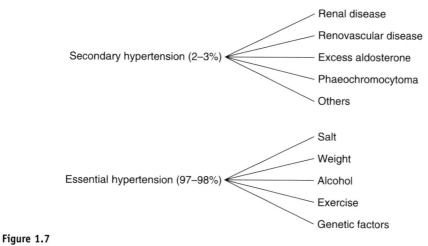

Figure 1.7
Essential and secondary hypertension.

Hypertension and the menopause

The overall prevalence of hypertension is estimated to be 30–50% in women aged 65 years or older. Indeed, hypertension is an important contributor to morbidity and mortality in postmenopausal women in western countries (Figure 1.8). Before the menopause, hypertension has a lower prevalence in women than in men, but beyond the age of 65 years, the mean systolic BP in women at least approaches that seen in older men, and has occasionally been reported to be even higher.

The exact underlying mechanisms responsible for this gender difference in BP are unclear, as is the influence of the menopause. Some longitudinal studies have not reported an independent increase of BP with the menopause. However, cross-sectional studies have found some pressor effect of the menopause on BP, independent of age and body mass index. Despite these conflicting data, it appears the 'dramatic' postmenopausal increase in BP might have additional or even other underlying causes than increasing age.

The lack of endogenous oestrogen production might play a major role in postmenopausal BP increase. Endothelium-dependent vasodilatation is also decreased in menopausal women, which is improved after administration of exogenous oestrogen, suggesting the involvement of oestrogen in BP regulation. Thus, oestrogen, or the lack of it, seems to be involved in the pathogenesis of the increase in postmenopausal BP.

> Hypertension rates are linked to the menopause, with lower prevalence in premenopausal women rising to rates similar to those of men in postmenopausal females. The exact mechanisms responsible for this remain unclear although the presence of oestrogen may be a factor

Further reading

1999 World Health Organisation – International Society Guidelines for the Management of Hypertension. Guidelines Subcommittee. *J Hypertens* 1999; **17**: 151–83.

Colhoun HM, Dong W, Poulter NR. Blood pressure screening, management and control in England: results from the health survey for England 1994. *J Hypertens* 1998; **16**: 747–52.

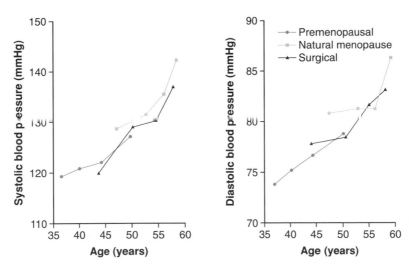

Figure 1.8
The influence of the menopause on blood pressure. The adjusted blood pressure rise with age was steeper in post-menopausal women. [Adapted from Staessen *et al*. *J Hum Hypertens* 1989; **3**: 427–33.]

Eastern Stroke and Coronary Heart Disease Collaborative Research Group. Blood pressure, cholesterol, and stroke in eastern Asia. *Lancet* 1998; **352**: 1801–7.

Ramsay L, Williams B, Johnston GD *et al.* Guidelines for management of hypertension: report of the third working party of the British Hypertension Society. *J Hum Hypertens* 1999; **13**: 569–92.

Rosenthal T, Oparil S. Hypertension in women. *J Hum Hypertens* 2000; **14**: 691–704.

Seedat YK. Hypertension in developing nations in sub-Saharan Africa. *J Hum Hypertens* 2000; **14**: 739–47.

Singh RB, Suh IL, Singh VP *et al.* Hypertension and stroke in Asia: prevalence, control and strategies in developing countries for prevention. *J Hum Hypertens* 2000; **14**: 749–63.

The sixth report of the Joint National Committee on prevention, detection, evaluation and treatment of high blood pressure. *Arch Intern Med* 1997; **157**: 2413–46.

Ueshima H, Zhang XH, Choudhury SR. Epidemiology of hypertension in China and Japan. *J Hum Hypertens* 2000; **14**: 765–9.

Wood D, Durrington P, Poulter N *et al.* Joint British recommendations on prevention of coronary heart disease in clinical practice. *Heart* 1998; **80(2)**: S1–29.

2. Pathophysiology

Cardiac output and peripheral resistance
Renin–angiotensin system
Autonomic nervous system
Hypercoagulability
Endothelial dysfunction
Other factors
Intrauterine influences

- low birth weight
- intrauterine nutrition
- neurovascular anomalies.

Their relative roles may differ between individuals and ethnic groups. For example, there is a high prevalence of insulin resistance in the peoples of South Asia which can be associated with obesity, diabetes and lipid abnormalities – the so-called 'metabolic syndrome'.

> Hypertension has a complex pathophysiology with most cases exhibiting no clear single identifiable cause, though abnormalities in the physiological mechanisms involved in maintaining normal BP may play a part in its development

The pathophysiology of hypertension is complex and is the subject of much uncertainty. In most cases (95%), no clear single identifiable cause is found and the condition is labelled 'essential hypertension'. A small number of patients (between 2% and 5%) have an underlying secondary disease as the cause of their hypertension.

Many physiological mechanisms are involved in the maintenance of normal blood pressure (BP), and pathophysiological abnormalities in these systems might play a part in the development of essential hypertension. The factors that influence BP include:

- salt intake
- obesity and insulin resistance
- the renin–angiotensin system
- sympathetic nervous system.

Additional factors proposed include:

- genetics
- endothelial dysfunction (including changes in mediators, such as endothelin and nitric oxide)
- hypercoagulability

Cardiac output and peripheral resistance

Normal BP depends upon a balance between the cardiac output and peripheral vascular resistance. In essential hypertension, cardiac output is normal but peripheral resistance is raised. The peripheral resistance is determined by the state of small arterioles, the walls of which contain smooth muscle cells, and not by the large arteries or the capillaries.

Moderate BP increase

With mild to moderate elevations in BP, the initial response of the vasculature is arterial and arteriolar vasoconstriction. Thus autoregulation maintains tissue perfusion at a relatively constant level and prevents the raised BP from damaging the smaller, more distal blood vessels. Prolonged smooth muscle constriction induces structural changes in these arterioles, with vessel wall thickening possibly mediated by angiotensin. This leads to an irreversible rise in peripheral resistance. The intracellular calcium concentration found in smooth muscle cells is responsible for this contraction. This explains the vasodilatory effect of calcium channel blockers.

Cause and effect of early hypertension

In very early hypertension, elevation of the BP may also be caused by a raised cardiac output related to sympathetic overactivity (peripheral resistance is not raised). Peripheral resistance subsequently rises in a compensatory manner to prevent the raised pressure being transmitted to the capillary bed where it would substantially affect cell homeostasis. The later arteriolar hypertrophy also minimizes the transmission of pressure to the capillary circulation.

> In very early hypertension, raised BP may be caused by a raised cardiac output related to sympathetic overactivity

Severe hypertension

In very severe hypertension, eg as seen in hypertensive emergencies, intense peripheral vasoconstriction takes place, resulting in:

- a rapid rise in BP
- ischaemia of the brain
- ischaemia of the peripheral organs.

This ischaemia stimulates neurohormone and cytokine release, exacerbating the vasoconstriction and ischaemia, further increasing the BP and leading to target organ damage. In addition, myointimal proliferation in the vasculature can make the situation worse, as may disseminated intravascular coagulation. Furthermore, renal ischaemia leads to the activation of the renin–angiotensin system, thereby causing a further rise in BP and microvascular damage.

With rapid and severe rises in BP, the process of autoregulation fails. This leads to a rise in pressure in the arterioles and capillaries and causes vascular damage. This disruption of the endothelium allows plasma constituents (including fibrinoid material) to enter the vessel wall, narrowing or obliterating the lumen in many tissue beds. The level at which fibrinoid necrosis occurs is dependent upon the baseline BP. In the cerebral circulation, this can lead to the development of cerebral oedema and the clinical picture of hypertensive encephalopathy.

In addition to protecting the tissues against the effects of hypertension, autoregulation maintains perfusion during the treatment of hypertension via arterial and arteriolar vasodilatation.

In chronic hypertension, autoregulation of cerebral blood flow is shifted towards higher BPs, with impairment of the tolerance to acute hypotension.

However, excessive falls in BP below the autoregulatory range can lead to organ ischaemia. The arteriolar hypertrophy induced by chronic hypertension means that target organ ischaemia will occur at a higher BP than in previously normotensive subjects.

As an example, in normotensive subjects, the upper limit of autoregulation can be a mean arterial pressure of 120 mmHg (or about 160/100 mmHg), but in individuals whose vessels are hypertrophied by longstanding hypertension, it may be substantially higher.

> Rapid and severe rises in BP can cause autoregulation to fail; this leads to vascular damage caused by a rise in pressure in the arterioles and capillaries

Renin–angiotensin system

The renin–angiotensin system is probably the most important of the endocrine systems controlling the BP. The kidney's juxtaglomerular apparatus secretes renin in response to glomerular underperfusion or a reduced salt intake. Renin is also released in response to stimulation from the sympathetic nervous system. Renin is responsible for converting renin substrate, angiotensinogen, to angiotensin I, a physiologically inactive substance. Angiotensin I is rapidly converted to angiotensin II in the lungs by angiotensin-converting enzyme (ACE). Angiotensin II is a potent vasoconstrictor and thus causes a rise in BP. It also stimulates the release of aldosterone from the adrenal zona glomerulosa, which results in both sodium and water retention (Figure 2.1).

There are also important non-circulating 'local' renin–angiotensin epicrine or paracrine systems

in the kidney, the heart and in the arterial tree. These also effect the BP and might have important roles in regulating regional blood flow.

Link with hypertension

While the circulating renin–angiotensin system is not thought to be directly responsible for the rise in BP in essential

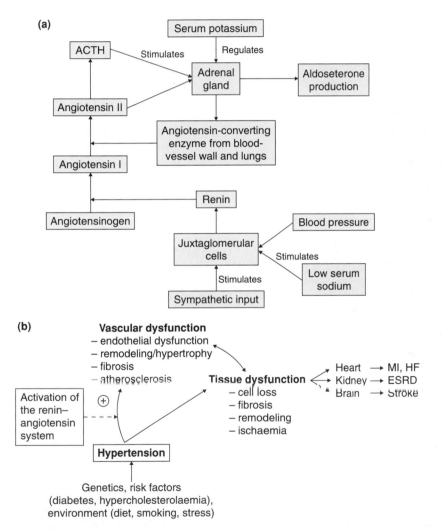

Figure 2.1
(a) The renin–angiotensin–aldosterone system; (b) The renin–angiotensin drives the pathology in hypertension. ESRD, end stage renal disease; HF, heart failure; MI, myocardial infarction. [Adapted from Weir *et al. Am J Hypertens* 1999; **12**: 205S–235; Timmermans *et al. Pharmacol Rev* 1993; **45**: 205–51.]

hypertension, many of the drugs we use for treating hypertension influence this endocrine system. Furthermore, many hypertensive patients have low levels of renin and angiotensin II (especially elderly and Afro-Caribbean people). Drugs that block the renin–angiotensin system are not particularly effective in these patient groups (Table 2.1).

Autonomic nervous system

The autonomic nervous system plays an important role in the pathophysiology of hypertension and is key to maintaining a normal BP. For example, sympathetic nervous system stimulation can cause both arteriolar constriction and arteriolar dilatation depending on whether or not the receptors are excitatory or inhibitory.

The autonomic nervous system is important in the mediation of short-term changes in BP in response to stress and physical exercise. However, adrenaline and noradrenaline may not have a clear role in the aetiology of hypertension; although drugs used for the treatment of hypertension do block the sympathetic nervous system and have a well-established therapeutic role. There is more likely to be a complex interaction between the autonomic nervous system and the various neuroendocrine systems, together with other factors, including circulating sodium volume.

> The autonomic nervous system has a central role in:
> - the pathophysiology of hypertension
> - maintaining a normal BP
> - mediating short term changes in BP in response to stress and physical exercise

Hypercoagulability

Although the blood vessels are exposed to high pressures in hypertension, paradoxically, the main complications of hypertension, stroke and myocardial infarction (MI) are thrombotic rather than haemorrhagic – the thrombotic paradox of hypertension. This is also known as the 'Birmingham paradox' (Figure 2.2). Increasing evidence suggests that patients with hypertension demonstrate:

- abnormalities of vessel walls (endothelial dysfunction or damage)
- abnormal levels of blood constituents (haemostatic factors, platelet activation and fibrinolysis)
- abnormal blood flow (rheology, viscosity and flow reserve).

The fulfilment of the three components of Virchow's triad for thrombogenesis suggests that hypertension confers a prothrombotic or hypercoagulable state, which appears to be related to the degree or severity of target organ damage. These abnormalities can be related to a long-term prognosis and may be altered by antihypertensive treatment.

Table 2.1
Drugs which block the renin system (beta-blockers, ACE inhibitors and angiotensin I receptor blockers) tend to be less effective in patients with low renin and angiotensin levels

- Low renin states
- Anephrics
- Conn's syndrome
- Liquorice-induced hypertension
- Older patients
- Afro-Caribbeans
- Type 2 diabetics

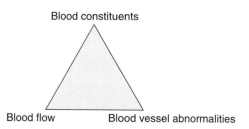

Figure 2.2
Virchow's triad of thrombogenesis. Abnormalities of all three components of Virchows triad are present in hypertension; hypertension confers a prothrombotic state.

Endothelial dysfunction

Vascular endothelial cells play a key role in cardiovascular regulation by producing a number of potent local vasoactive agents, including the vasodilator molecule nitric oxide (NO) and the vasoconstrictor peptide endothelin. Dysfunction of the endothelium has been implicated in human essential hypertension.

Modulation of the endothelial function is an attractive therapeutic option in attempting to minimize some of the important complications of hypertension. Clinically effective antihypertensive therapy appears to restore impaired production of NO, but does not seem to restore the impaired endothelium-dependent vascular relaxation or vascular response to endothelial receptors. This indicates that such endothelial dysfunction is primary and becomes irreversible once the hypertensive process has become established.

Vasoactive substances

Many vasoactive systems and mechanisms that affect sodium transport and vascular tone are involved in maintaining normal BP:

- Endothelin is a powerful, vascular, endothelial vasoconstrictor which may produce a 'salt sensitive' rise in BP. It also activates local renin–angiotensin systems.
- Bradykinin is a potent vasodilator, which is inactivated by an angiotensin-converting enzyme. Consequently, treatment with ACE inhibitors may exert some of their effect by blocking bradykinin inactivation.
- Endothelial-derived relaxant factor, which is now known to be NO is produced by arterial and venous endothelium and diffuses through the vessel wall into the smooth muscle causing vasodilatation. Nevibilol, a new generation beta-blocker, also has NO-modulating effects, although its full clinical impact is still uncertain. However, it is possible that this property may mean it causes fewer side-effects than other beta-blockers, eg does not cause impotence.

- Atrial natriuretic peptide (ANP) is a hormone secreted from the atria of the heart in response to increased blood volume. The effect of ANP is to increase sodium and water excretion from the kidney. Modulation of this hormone, with the aim of treating hypertension and heart failure, has been a target of new agents such as omapatrilat, a vasopeptidase inhibitor, but further data are awaited.

> Many vasoactive systems and sodium transport-affecting mechanisms are involved in maintaining normal BP, such as endothelin and bradykinin

Other factors

Angiogenesis

Abnormal angiogenesis has been demonstrated in animal models of hypertension as well as in different stages of hypertension in humans. In hypertension, there seems to be an impaired ability for vascular growth resulting from structural alteration of the microvascular network. This includes capillary rarefaction and increased arteriolar length and tortuosity. These alterations in the microvasculature appear at very early stages of hypertension and increasing evidence points to the possibility that abnormal angiogenesis may contribute causally to hypertension.

Sodium transport

The transport of sodium across vascular smooth muscle cell walls could influence the BP through its relationship with calcium transport.

Insulin sensitivity

Several 'classic' risk factors tend to go together leading to the suggestion that these represent a single syndrome (the so-called 'metabolic syndrome X' or Reaven's syndrome). These factors include:

- obesity
- glucose intolerance
- diabetes mellitus
- hyperlipidaemia.

This syndrome causes raised BP, vascular damage and marked cardiovascular risk. However, some hypertensive patients who are not obese also display resistance to insulin. The metabolic syndrome, which appears to be prevalent in South Asians who are at high risk of ischaemic heart disease, could explain why the hazards of cardiovascular risk are synergistic or multiplicative rather than simply additive.

Genetic factors

Human essential hypertension is a complex, multifactorial, quantitative trait under polygenic control. Over the last decade several strategies have been used to dissect the genetic determinants of hypertension. Separate genes and genetic factors have been linked to the development of essential hypertension, but many genes probably contribute to the development of the disorder in any particular individual. It is rare that one specific genetic mutation can cause hypertension and the condition is twice as common in subjects with one or two hypertensive parents. Genetic factors account for approximately 30% of the variation in BP in various populations.

In the quest for a gene (or genes) for hypertension, the study of rare monogenic forms of hypertension has been the most successful. Attempts to identify the multiple genes involved in the more common polygenic form of hypertension has been much more difficult. Many laboratories use rat models of genetic hypertension so some of the complexity of studying human hypertension can be removed, but whether such information can be applied to large populations of hypertensive humans is debatable. Numerous crosses between hypertensive and normotensive rat strains have produced several quantitative trait loci for:

- blood pressure
- left ventricular hypertrophy
- stroke
- insulin resistance
- kidney failure.

Rural vs urban populations

While hypertension is pretty rare in rural or 'tribal' areas of Africa, it is very common in African cities and in Afro-Caribbean populations in the UK and the USA. The rural/urban differences in Africa may be due to lifestyle and dietary factors, but the discovery that hypertension is more common in Afro-Caribbeans than in Caucasians may have a genetic basis.

Intrauterine influences

Fetal influences, particularly birth weight, may be a determinant of BP in adult life, although the precise pathophysiological mechanisms are still uncertain. For example, babies with a small birth weight are more likely to have higher BPs during adolescence and to be hypertensive as adults.

The Barker hypothesis states that small-for-age babies are also more likely to have metabolic abnormalities, which have been associated with the later development of hypertension and cardiovascular disease. These metabolic abnormalities include:

- insulin resistance
- diabetes mellitus
- hyperlipidaemia
- abdominal obesity.

Another interpretation suggests that genetic factors may explain the Barker hypothesis. For example, mothers with above average BP during pregnancy give birth to smaller babies who subsequently develop above average BP themselves and eventually hypertension. It is entirely likely that the similarity of BPs in mother and child are genetic, and in a modern 'healthy' society, BPs are unrelated to intrauterine under-nutrition.

Further reading

Blann AD, Lip GYH. The endothelium in atherothrombotic disease: assessment of function, mechanisms and clinical implications. *Blood Coagul Fibrinolysis* 1998; **9**: 297–306.

Eriksson JG, Forsen T, Tuomilehto J et al. Early growth and coronary heart disease in later life: longitudinal study. BMJ 2001; **322**: 949–53.

Gibbons GH. The pathophysiology of hypertension: the importance of angiotensin II in cardiovascular remodeling. Am J Hypertens 1998; **11**: 177S–181S.

Lee WK, Padmanabhan S, Dominiczak AF. Genetics of hypertension: from experimental models to clinical applications. J Hum Hypertens 2000; **14**: 631–47.

Le Noble FA, Stassen FR, Hacking WJ, Struijker Boudier HA. Angiogenesis and hypertension. J Hypertens 1998; **16**: 1563–72.

Lip GYH. Hypertension and the prothrombotic state. J Hum Hypertens 2000; **14**: 687–90.

Lip GYH, Blann AD. Does hypertension confer a prothrombotic state? Virchow's triad revisited. Circulation 2000; **101**: 218–20.

Nicholls MG, Robertson JI. The renin–angiotensin system in the year 2000. J Hum Hypertens 2000; **14**: 649–66.

Roseboom TJ, van der Meulen JH, van Montfrans GA et al. Maternal nutrition during gestation and blood pressure in later life. J Hypertens 2001; **19**: 29–34.

Ross R. The pathogenesis of atherosclerosis: a perspective for the 1990s. Nature 1993; **362**: 801–9.

Sagnella GA. Atrial natriuretic peptide mimetics and vasopeptidase inhibitors. Cardiovasc Res 2001; **51**: 416–28.

Schlaich MP, Schmieder RE. Left ventricular hypertrophy and its regression: pathophysiology and therapeutic approach: focus on treatment by antihypertensive agents. Am J Hypertens 1998; **11**: 1394–404.

Spieker LE, Noll G, Ruschitzka FT et al. Working under pressure: the vascular endothelium in arterial hypertension. J Hum Hypertens 2000; **14**: 617–30.

3. Target organ damage

Cerebrovascular disease
Heart
Large vessel arterial disease
Kidney and renal failure
Retinopathy
Hypertension in the context of overall risk

Table 3.1
Definite and possible risk factors for stroke

Definite	Possible
Hypertension	Lipid level
Artial fibrillation	Salt consumption
Coronary heart disease	Low K+ diet
NIDDM	Low Vitamin C diet
TIA	Fibrinogen
Smoking	
Carotid disease	
Alcohol excess	

NIDDM, non insulin-dependent diabetis mellitus; TIA, transient ischaemic attack

The natural history of high blood pressure (BP) can be regarded as having two stages:

- Initially, hypertension can develop as a risk factor, without significant local organ damage or symptoms.
- Later, this can shift towards significant target organ damage with cardiovascular symptoms. This can manifest itself as blocking effects (atherothrombotic plaques causing coronary, cerebrovascular or peripheral artery disease) or bursting effects (cerebral haemorrhage, aortic dissection or heart failure).

Cerebrovascular disease

Stroke is one of the most devastating consequences of hypertension, resulting not only in premature death, but also in significant disability. Definite and possible stroke risk factors are summarized in Table 3.1.

Strokes account for about 12% of all deaths and about 25% of all strokes occur in patients younger than 65 years. After standardizing for age, men aged 40–59 years with a systolic BP of 160–180 mmHg are approximately four times more likely to suffer a stroke during the next eight years when compared to men with a

systolic BP of 140–159 mmHg. An average reduction of just 9/5 mmHg in BP results in a 34% reduction in the incidence of stroke whereas a reduction of 19/10 mmHg results in a 56% lower incidence of stroke.

Strokes account for 12% of all deaths. 25% of all strokes affect the under 65 age group; men with a systolic BP of 160–180 mmHg are around four times more likely to have a stroke than men with a BP of 140–159 mmHg

In patients with hypertension, about 80% of strokes are ischaemic. They are caused by intra-arterial thrombosis or embolization from the heart and large arteries. The remaining 20% are due to haemorrhagic causes, which may also be related to very high BP. In the UK, 40% of all strokes are estimated to be linked to a systolic BP of ≥140 mmHg. The relationship between prior blood pressure control and odds ratio for stroke is illustrated in Figure 3.1. Stroke recurrence after TIA or minor stroke is also greater with higher blood pressures (see Figure 3.2).

Strokes and the elderly

Elderly hypertensive patients are particularly prone to developing all types of stroke and often sustain multiple small asymptomatic cerebral infarcts, leading to progressive loss of intellectual function and dementia. Indeed, the recent Syst–Eur study convincingly showed that treatment of isolated systolic hypertension, which is more frequently seen in the elderly, resulted in the prevention of dementia at follow-up (Table 3.2).

Strokes and atrial fibrillation

Hypertension is also associated with an increased risk of atrial fibrillation, which is the most common sustained cardiac rhythm disorder. The presence of both hypertension and atrial fibrillation increases the risk of stroke. In the low-risk arm of the third Stroke Prevention in Atrial Fibrillation study (SPAF-3), even a previous history of hypertension increased the risk of stroke nearly four-fold, despite aspirin therapy.

Heart

Coronary heart disease

Fatal coronary heart disease (CHD) is seven times more common among hypertensives than a fatal stroke, and is the major population consequence of hypertension. Controlled trials have consistently shown that treating high BP can largely prevent stroke and heart failure, but the reduction of coronary thrombosis is less

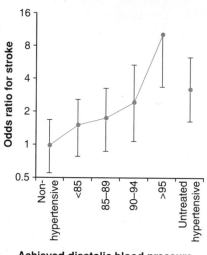

Achieved diastolic blood pressure (mmHg) in past 5 years

Figure 3.1
Prior blood pressure control and odds ratio for stroke
[Adapted from Du *et al. Br Med J* 1997; **314**: 272–6.]

Table 3.2
The Syst-Eur dementia sub-study

	Placebo	Active	
Number in trial	1180	1238	
All dementia	21	11	*p*<0.05
Alzheimer's	15	8	NS
Mixed	4	3	NS
Vascular	2	0	NS

[Adapted from Forette *et al. Lancet* 1998; **352**: 1347–51]

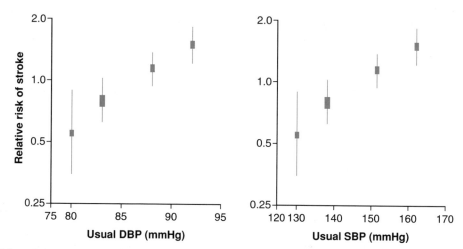

Figure 3.2
Stroke recurrence after TIA or minor stroke. DBP, diastolic blood pressure; SBP, systolic blood pressure. [Adapted from Rogers *et al. Br Med J* 1996; **313**: 147.]

impressive. Nevertheless, analysis of the large treatment trials suggests that adequate treatment of hypertension reduces the risk of heart attack by approximately 25% (although this is based on BP reduction with thiazides and beta-blockers, rather than the newer antihypertensive drugs).

Left ventricular hypertrophy

As a result of the increased pressure against which the heart has to pump blood, the mass of the left ventricular muscle increases. While this is initially a compensatory response, increased muscle mass eventually outstrips its oxygen supply. When left ventricular hypertrophy (LVH) is coupled with the reduced coronary vascular reserve seen in hypertension, it can result in myocardial ischaemia even with normal coronary arteries.

Thus, beyond a certain point, LVH secondary to hypertension becomes a major risk factor for:

- myocardial infarction
- stroke
- congestive cardiac failure
- sudden death.

This increased risk is in addition to that imposed by hypertension itself. Hypertensives with LVH are also at an increased risk of developing cardiac arrhythmias (atrial fibrillation, ventricular arrhythmias) and atherosclerotic vascular disease (coronary and peripheral artery disease).

If LVH is present, the prognosis for cardiac failure and stroke is three or four times worse for any given BP.

Pathogenesis

The mechanisms promoting the development of LVH remain uncertain. The basic underlying mechanism may be an increase in ventricular wall stress and pressure workload on the left ventricle. Thus, with an increase in afterload as a result of hypertension, the heart responds with an increase in wall thickness. There is, however, a poor correlation between left ventricular wall thickness and BP. In addition, the pathogenesis of LVH has been shown to be influenced by:

- demographic factors, eg age, sex, race and body habitus
- exogenous factors, eg dietary salt intake and alcohol consumption
- neurohumoral substances, eg activity of the renin–angiotensin–aldosterone system, the sympathetic system, growth hormone and insulin.

Several mechanisms have also been postulated for the role of the renin–angiotensin system in the pathogenesis of LVH:

- First, angiotensin II has direct and widespread vasoconstrictor properties, affecting left ventricular afterload and myocardial ischaemia.
- Second, angiotensin II can also indirectly stimulate myocyte hypertrophy via its interaction with sympathetic tone and in addition could be trophic to myocytes. This may stimulate fibroblastic proliferation and collagen formation; these factors are involved in the development of LVH (Table 3.3).

> The factors affecting the development of LVH remain unclear. The basic underlying mechanism may be an increase in ventricular wall stress and pressure workload on the left ventricle

Table 3.3
Possible adverse features of left ventricular hypertrophy

- Mismatch of blood supply and non-vascular tissue resulting in a relatively 'starved' subendocardial region
- Increased basal myocardial oxygen demand due to increased mass and wall stress
- A heightened likelihood of ventricular arrhythmias, perhaps related to the presence of fibrous tissue
- A markedly reduced coronary flow reserve, with abnormalities in the ability to dilate coronary arteries, resulting in increased cardiac ischaemia

Screening

A commonly used screening test for LVH in hypertensive patients is the 12-lead electrocardiogram (ECG). The usual criteria are those proposed by Sokolow and Lyon, that is, the sum of the S wave in lead V1 and the R wave in leads V5 or V6 on the ECG must be >35 mm. Nevertheless, LVH can be identified by electrocardiography in only 5–10% of hypertensive patients. Echocardiography is a far more sensitive investigation, identifying LVH in around 50% of untreated hypertensive patients. The various ECG criteria used for defining LVH are summarized in Table 3.4.

Cardiac arrhythmia

LVH is also a risk factor for the development of cardiac arrhythmias, the most common being atrial fibrillation and ventricular arrhythmias. The presence of atrial fibrillation is important as this arrhythmia is associated with a five-fold increase in mortality and may often require long-term antiarrhythmic and antithrombotic therapy. Ventricular arrhythmias also have important implications for the risk of sudden death in these patients. The mechanisms for sudden death are complex and may include malignant cardiac arrhythmias, such as increased ventricular ectopics and nonsustained ventricular tachycardia. However, this risk of sudden death is independent of arterial pressure. Electrophysiological mechanisms for arrhythmogenesis in LVH are summarized in Table 3.5.

> LVH is a risk factor for developing cardiac arrhythmias, such as atrial fibrillation (which is associated with a five-fold increase in mortality) and ventricular arrhythmias

Heart failure as a complication of LVH

Heart failure is another complication commonly associated with LVH and hypertension. The way hypertension results in heart failure is unclear, but may occur as a result of pressure overload, for example the excessive demand of afterload on an otherwise normal heart. LVH may also result in:

- impaired cardiac function that is secondary to diastolic dysfunction
- subendocardial ischaemia
- an inefficient cardiac rhythm due to frequent arrhythmias or even atrial fibrillation.

Table 3.5
Electrophysiological mechanisms for arrhythmogenesis in left ventricular hypertrophy

- Re-entry mechanisms related to myocardial fibrosis in left ventricular hypertrophy
- Myocardial ischaemic areas, perhaps related to reduced coronary reserve (as coronary artery disease is often not present)
- Ventricular myocyte stretching and arterial wall tension in the hypertrophied heart
- Increased sympathetic nervous system activity

Table 3.4
Electrocardiographic criteria for the diagnosis of left ventricular hypertrophy

Criterion	Measurement	Author(s) and year of description
R wave in aVL	R aVL	Sokolow and Lyon 1949
Sokolow-Lyon	SV1 + R(V5 or V6)	Sokolow and Lyon 1949
Cornell	RaVL + SV3	Casale et al. 1985
Cornell Voltage Duration Product	RaVL + SV3 × QRS duration	Molloy et al. 1992
Cornell / QRS II	RaVL + SV3/Total QRS voltage in lead II	Denarié et al. 1998
Lewis	RI – RIII + SIII – SI	Lewis 1914
RI + SIII	RI + SIII	Gubner & Ungerleider 1943

A final mechanism is the association with coronary artery disease, which may result in cardiac ischaemia (with ventricular impairment or 'hibernation') or myocardial infarction (Figure 3.3).

Antihypertensive drugs

It should be emphasized that LVH is preventable by using antihypertensive medication and improving control of hypertension. In fact, almost every antihypertensive drug is capable of reducing cardiac mass and reversing LVH if therapy is maintained for long enough. The reduction in left ventricular mass also correlates with the reduction in mean arterial pressure.

Not all antihypertensive drugs result in the regression of LVH in a similar fashion. For example, angiotensin-converting enzyme (ACE) inhibitors appear more effective in the regression of LVH than beta-blockers and diuretics (Figure 3.4). By contrast, directly acting vasodilators, such as minoxidil and hydralazine, have little impact on LVH.

The effects of left ventricular mass reduction often run parallel with the reduction in BP as a result of treatment. There is also evidence that

cardiac arrhythmias, myocardial ischaemia and impaired ventricular filling diminish in parallel to the reduction in left ventricular mass and the regression of LVH. In the Framingham study, patients with a reduction in LVH showed a

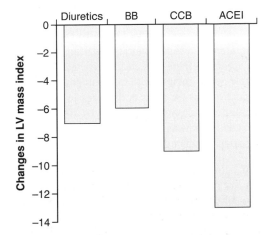

Figure 3.4
Reversal of left ventricular hypertrophy in essential hypertension – meta analysis data showing changes in left ventricular mass index with different classes of antihypertensive agent. BB, beta-blocker; CCB, calcium channel blockers; ACEI, angiotensin-converting enzyme inhibitors. [Adapted from Schmeider *et al. JAMA* 1996; **275:** 1507–13.]

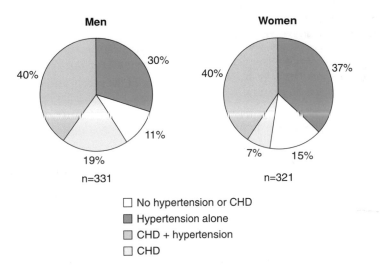

Figure 3.3
Prevalence of coronary heart disease and hypertension in chronic heart failure as seen in the Framingham Heart study. CHD, coronary heart disease.

decrease of at least 25% in cardiovascular mortality over four years, the effect being most beneficial in men.

In the recent Losartan Intervention for Endpoint Reduction in Hypertension (LIFE) trial in high-risk patients with essential hypertension and ECG evidence of LVH, the primary composite endpoint was reduced by 13% with the angiotensin receptor blocker losartan compared to atenolol. There was also a 25% reduction in stroke when treated with losartan and a 25% reduction in new cases of diabetes in patients treated with losartan compared to atenolol. Indeed, there was more regression of LVH with losartan compared to atenolol.

> Not all antihypertensive drugs operate in the same way to reduce LVH; for example, ACE inhibitors appear to be more effective than beta-blockers and diuretics, while directly acting vasodilators have little impact

Heart failure

Convincing evidence from prospective epidemiological studies suggests that heart failure can be caused by high BP and may be prevented by its control. For example, the Framingham study suggested that high BP was the principal cause of heart failure; subjects with BP >160/95 mmHg had a six-fold higher incidence of heart failure than those with BP <140/90 mmHg. Heart failure has a poor long-term prognosis. The New York Heart Association (NYHA) Grade IV Heart failure has a worse prognosis than cancer, with a one-year mortality of over 50%. Heart failure in association with untreated hypertension can, over many years, slowly be replaced by 'normal' BP as the left ventricular muscle progressively fails.

In the Framingham study it was shown that the presence of LVH on the ECG substantially increases the risk of heart failure. Hypertension increases the risk of CHD and subsequent myocardial infarction (MI) – the most common cause of heart failure in the UK. Hypertension contributes to the development of atrial

fibrillation; and if hypertensive LVH and diastolic dysfunction are present, the sudden onset of atrial fibrillation can precipitate acute heart failure. Finally, hypertension in association with renal artery stenosis can cause 'flash' pulmonary oedema. This condition can be corrected by treatment of the renal artery stenosis.

Diastolic dysfunction

In hypertensive LVH, the ventricle cannot relax normally during diastole. Thus, to produce the necessary increase in ventricular input, especially during exercise, there is an increase in left atrial pressure rather than the normal reduction in ventricular pressure. This can lead to an elevation in pulmonary capillary pressure that is sufficient to induce pulmonary congestion. The rise in atrial pressure can also lead to atrial fibrillation. In hypertrophied ventricles dependent upon atrial systole, the loss of atrial transport can result in a significant reduction in stroke volume and pulmonary oedema. Exercise-induced subendocardial ischaemia can produce 'exaggerated' impairment of diastolic relaxation of the hypertrophied myocardium.

Large vessel arterial disease

Peripheral vascular disease (PVD) is associated with high cardiovascular morbidity and mortality. Intermittent claudication:

- is the most common symptomatic manifestation of PVD
- is an important predictor of cardiovascular death – increasing it three-fold
- increases all-cause mortality by between two and five times.

Hypertension is a common and important risk factor for vascular disorders, including PVD. About 2–5% of hypertensive patients have intermittent claudication at presentation and the prevalence increases with age. Similarly, 35–55% of patients with PVD at presentation also have hypertension. Patients who suffer from hypertension with PVD have a greatly increased risk of MI and stroke. Many patients with PVD also have renal artery stenosis, which is often unsuspected (Figure 3.5). This may also contribute to their hypertension

> The most common symptom of PVD is intermittent claudication. Intermittent claudication also causes a three-fold increase in the chance of cardiovascular death

Atherogenesis

Atheromatous disease in the aorta coupled with hypertension may progress to aortic aneurysm, the majority of which occur in hypertensive patients. High pulsatile wave stress and atheromatous disease can lead to dissection of the aorta, which carries a high short-term mortality. Extracranial carotid artery disease is also more common in hypertensive patients and is one of the mechanisms by which hypertension leads to the increased risk of stroke.

Apart from the epidemiological associations, hypertension also contributes to the pathogenesis of atherosclerosis – the basic pathological process underlying PVD. Hypertension is associated with abnormalities of haemostasis and of blood lipids (as is PVD), leading to an increased atherothrombotic state. None of the large treatment trials have adequately addressed whether or not a reduction in BP causes a decrease in PVD incidence. There is an obvious need for such outcome studies to correlate the effect of BP reduction on the incidence of PVD, especially since the two

conditions are commonly encountered together, but the association is often forgotten.

> The majority of aortic aneurysms occur in hypertensive patients, where high pulsatile wave stress and atheromatous disease can result in dissection of the aorta

Kidney and renal failure

Renal dysfunction is often found in hypertensive patients and malignant hypertension frequently leads to progressive renal failure. There is some controversy as to whether or not mild-to-moderate essential hypertension leads to renal failure. It may be that patients who develop renal failure actually have hypertension secondary to renal disease, rather than vice versa.

In the Renfrew community project, individuals with raised BP had a higher frequency of left ventricular enlargement (as seen on ECG) assessed by the Minnesota code and slightly larger cardiothoracic ratios on chest X-ray. In sharp contrast, serum creatinine, as an index of renal damage, did not differ when comparing hypertensive patients to normotensive patients. If, like LVH, serum creatinine is an index of target organ damage in hypertension, then higher serum creatinine levels would be expected in hypertensive patients. Thus the relationship between hypertension and the kidney is qualitatively rather than quantitatively different from the link between hypertension and cardiac or cerebral damage.

Proteinuria

In hypertensive patients, the presence of proteinuria is prognostically important and is associated with a roughly two-fold increase in cardiovascular mortality. Microproteinuria has been considered to be evidence of early BP-induced kidney damage. Relationships have been found between microproteinuria and the left ventricular mass on echocardiography.

In the International study of Salt and Blood Pressure (INTERSALT) project, no relationship

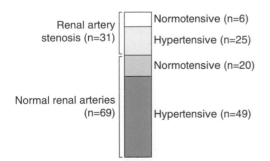

Figure 3.5
Renal artery stenosis in peripheral vascular disease
[Adapted from Wachtell et al. J Hum Hypertens 1996; **10**: 83–5.]

was found between the height of the systolic or diastolic BP and the amount of protein in urine. It is important to remember that protein can leak into the urine due to non-BP related causes where there is unequivocally no damage to the nephron. These conditions include:

- fever
- heart failure
- changes in posture
- vigorous exercise
- trauma
- burns.

There are no reported cases of benign essential hypertensive patients with normal serum creatinine levels and no proteinuria who subsequently went on to develop renal failure. This is in sharp contrast to the relationship between hypertension and its cardiovascular and cerebral complications, where uncomplicated benign hypertension frequently leads to the development of heart attacks or strokes. These data strongly suggest that only those patients with primary renal disease will progress to develop end-stage renal failure (Figure 3.6).

Possible mechanisms of renal damage

Several hormones, some of which have a renal origin, are involved in the maintenance of BP, renal blood flow and renal function. Most of these mechanisms explain why kidney diseases cause raised BP rather vice versa. Some patients with hypertension-induced atheromatous disease of their renal arteries might be expected to develop renal impairment but that is not due to intrinsic kidney damage.

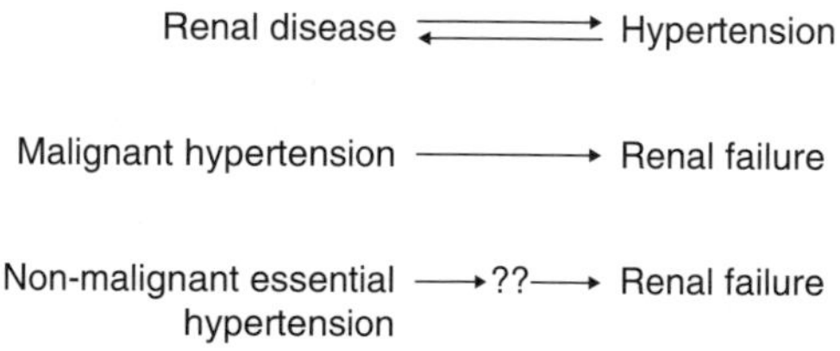

Renal disease ⟷ Hypertension

Malignant hypertension ⟶ Renal failure

Non-malignant essential ⟶??⟶ Renal failure
      hypertension

Figure 3.6
Hypertension and the kidney – the development of end stage renal failure.

Other possible mechanisms include nephro-toxicity of cardiovascular drugs, eg:

- a reduction of cardiac output and renal blood flow due to beta-blockade
- a reduction of renal plasma flow in patients treated with ACE inhibitors while in a state of intravascular volume depletion.

The vast majority of these patients with benign essential hypertension will not develop any renal damage whether they are treated or untreated.

> Several hormones made in the kidney help maintain BP, renal blood flow and renal functions, thereby explaining why kidney diseases cause raised BP rather than vice versa

Evidence from treatment trials

Among hypertensive patients, renal damage is rare compared to heart attacks and strokes, and the number of renal events encountered in the randomized treatment trials is very small. There is a definite lack of difference in renal endpoints in treated versus untreated hypertensive patients, with a tiny number of cases developing renal impairment.

Participants in the MRC trial of mild hypertension (including a cohort from Renfrew) had their serum urea levels measured at baseline and were restudied after three years; there was no difference at the outset between those patients who were randomized either to placebo, propranolol or bendrofluazide (bendroflumethiazide) treatment (Figure 3.7). A tendency to develop a rise in serum creatinine has been noted in African Americans with hypertension. However, it was striking that the relationship between BP and subsequent renal impairment was very weak compared with the close relationship between BP and the subsequent development of heart attack and strokes.

> Limited evidence exists that controlling BP in non-malignant essential hypertension influences renal function

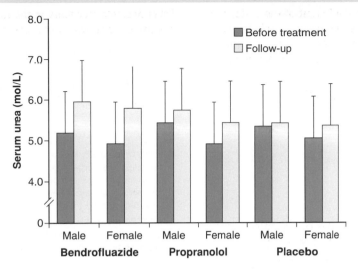

Figure 3.7
Changes in blood urea levels over five years. Data are from the Medical Research Council (MRC) trial. [Adapted from MRC Working Party on Mild Hypertension. *Br Med J* 1986; **293**: 988–92.]

Retinopathy

Hypertension leads to vascular changes in the eye, referred to as hypertensive retinopathy. These changes have been classified by Keith, Wagener and Barker into four grades; each grade correlates with a prognosis (Tables 3.6 and 3.7). Malignant hypertension, the most severe form, is clinically defined as raised BP in association with bilateral retinal flame-shaped haemorrhages and/or cotton wool spots and/or hard exudates, with or without papilloedema.

Hypertension in the context of overall risk

It must be remembered that hypertension is only one of a number of major risk factors for

Table 3.6
The Keith, Wagener, Barker classification

Grade I	Grade II	Grade III	Grade IV
• Benign hypertension	• More marked hypertensive retinopathy	• Mild angiospastic retinopathy	• Malignant hypertension
• Mild narrowing or sclerosis of the retinal arterioles	• Moderate to marked sclerosis of the retinal arterioles	• Retinal oedema, cotton-wool spots and haemorrhages	• All the features in Grades I–III plus optic disc oedema
• No symptoms	• Exaggerated arterial light reflex	• Sclerosis and spastic lesions of retinal arterioles	• Cardiac and renal functions may be impaired
• Good general health	• Venous compression at arterio-venous crossings	• Blood pressure often high and sustained	• Reduced survival
	• Blood pressure higher and more sustained than Group 1	• (Symptomatic)	
	• (Asymptomatic)		
	• Good general health		

Table 3.7
Keith, Wagener, Barker classification – patient survival

Years follow-up	Patient survival (%)			
	Grade I	Grade II	Grade III	Grade IV
1	90	88	65	21
3	70	62	22	6
5	70	54	20	1

[Adapted from Keith NM, Wagener HP, Barker NW. *Am J Med Sci* 1939; 196: 332–43]

CVD and strokes. The aim of treatment must be to prevent the complications of hypertension by reducing the BP to normal levels and detecting and correcting other cardiovascular risk factors.

Thus, when considering the individual patient, it is vital to take other risk factors such as smoking and diabetes into account. In the presence of risk factors, treating BP alone is relatively ineffective at preventing strokes and myocardial infarction (Table 3.8).

> Hypertension is only one of several major risk factors for CVD and strokes, and treating BP alone in the presence of risk factors is relatively ineffective

The treatment of hypertension is an almost unique therapeutic exercise. This is because large numbers of asymptomatic individuals are exposed to many years of treatment to prevent

potential adverse events in the future. In the context of the latest British recommendations for CVD prevention, the target BP is <140/90 mmHg (or even lower in some high-risk groups). As far as possible this should be carried out without causing the patient adverse physical effects from medication or other interventions.

Further reading

Dahlof B, Devereux RB, Kjeldsen SE *et al*. Cardiovascular morbidity and mortality in the Losartan Intervention For Endpoint reduction in hypertension study (LIFE): a randomised trial against atenolol. *Lancet* 2002; **359**: 995–1003.

Dahlof B, Pennert K, Hansson L. Reversal of left ventricular hypertrophy in hypertensive patients. A metaanalysis of 109 treatment studies. *Am J Hypertens* 1992; **5**: 95–110.

Levy D, Anderson KM, Savage DD *et al*. Echocardiographically detected left ventricular hypertrophy: prevalence and risk factors. The Framingham Heart Study. *Ann Intern Med* 1988; **108**: 7–13.

Lip GYH, Felmeden DC, Li-Saw-Hee FL, Beevers DG. Hypertensive heart disease. A complex syndrome or a hypertensive 'cardiomyopathy'? *Eur Heart J* 2000; **21**: 1653–65.

Rigaud AS, Seux ML, Staessen JA *et al*. Cerebral complications of hypertension. *J Hum Hypertens* 2000; **14**: 605–16.

Schmieder RE, Martus P, Klingbeil A. Reversal of left ventricular hypertrophy in essential hypertension. A meta-analysis of randomized double-blind studies. *JAMA* 1996; **275**: 1507–13.

Schmieder RE, Messerli FH. Hypertension and the heart. *J Hum Hypertens* 2000; **14**: 597–604.

Schmieder RE, Schlaich MP, Klingbeil AU, Martus P. Update on reversal of left ventricular hypertrophy in essential hypertension (a meta-analysis of all randomized double-blind studies until December 1996). *Nephrol Dial Transplant* 1998; **13**: 564–69.

Table 3.8
Hypertension risk factors

Risk factors	Target organ damage	Overt cardiovascular disease
Age	Left ventricular hypertrophy	Myocardial infarction
Gender	Proteinuria	Angina
Family history	Carotid atherosclerosis	Heart failure
Smoking	Diabetic nephropathy	PTCA/CABG
High serum cholesterol	Renal failure	Stroke/transient ischaemic attacks
Diabetes	Symptomatic arterial disease	
Obesity	Hypertensive retinopathy	

PTCA, percutaneous transluminal coronary angioplasty; CABG, coronary artery bypass graft surgery

4. Clinical assessment

Confirmation of the diagnosis
Investigations for all hypertensive patients
Investigations for selected patients
Blood pressure measurement

The management of the hypertensive patient (Table 4.1) requires:

- confirmation of the diagnosis
- assessment of the patient for the underlying cause(s) and target organ damage
- initiation of an appropriate therapy.

Confirmation of the diagnosis

The most important aspect of the management of a patient presenting with high blood pressure (BP) is to confirm the diagnosis of hypertension. Multiple measurements of BP over a period of time may show that BP levels fall over time so that a significant number of patients can no longer be regarded as

---

Table 4.1
Assessment of hypertensive patients

- Causes of hypertension, eg renal disease, endocrine causes
- Contributory factors, eg obesity, salt intake, excess alcohol intake
- Complications of hypertension, eg previous stroke, left ventricular hypertrophy
- Cardiovascular risk factors, eg smoking, family history
- Contraindications to specific drugs, eg asthma (beta-blockers), gout (thiazides)

---

hypertensive. Some patients develop high BP in relation to hospital or clinic attendance, the so-called 'white-coat' effect. Patients with 'white-coat' hypertension do not need antihypertensive therapy but do need careful monitoring as these patients may exhibit minor vascular changes and eventually develop overt hypertension in the future. Ambulatory BP monitoring devices have assisted the diagnosis of this condition. These monitors show the typical high BPs when the patient is attending the doctor/hospital and virtually normal BPs when the patient is relaxed at home.

It is a fundamental error to condemn a patient to decades of medication on only one or two casual BP measurements. Except for hypertensive emergencies or those in high-risk groups (including those exhibiting hypertensive target organ damage), it is good practice to take multiple BP readings over a few months while pursuing non-pharmacological measures before starting the patient on drug therapy.

> Multiple measurements of BP are advisable to diagnose hypertension, as a prelude to drug treatments. This helps avoid the misdiagnosis of 'white-coat' hypertension

Initial assessment

Each new patient requires a thorough clinical assessment, which should include a full cardiovascular examination. The basic investigations should include:

- blood biochemistry for urea and electrolytes, serum creatinine, fasting glucose and cholesterol
- urinalysis for blood, protein and glucose
- electrocardiogram (ECG).

Table 4.2 indicates the different tests that should be carried out. In some individuals, further investigations such as an echocardiogram or renal ultrasound may be required.

A chest X-ray, urine microscopy and culture and echocardiography are not routinely required. An

Table 4.2
Routine investigations in hypertensive patients

- Urine strip test, eg for protein and blood, which may indicate underlying renal disease
- Serum creatinine and electrolytes, which may raise a clinical suspicion of renal disease, Conn's syndrome etc
- Blood glucose, eg for associated diabetes
- Total serum cholesterol:HDL-cholesterol, which would allow associated hyperlipidaemia to be treated as part of overall cardiovascular risk prevention
- ECG, eg for diagnosis of associated rhythm abnormalities, myocardial infarction, LVH etc

echocardiogram is valuable to confirm or refute the presence of left ventricular hypertrophy (LVH) – when the ECG shows 'high' left ventricular voltage without T-wave abnormalities, as is often the case in young patients.

The primary purpose of the assessment is to exclude secondary causes of hypertension (Table 4.3) which, although accounting for fewer than 5% of hypertensive patients, are important to identify as they are often either correctable or may indicate a serious underlying disease. The majority of secondary causes are either renal, endocrine or due to concomitant medication, such as oestrogen-containing contraceptive pills or non-steroidal anti-inflammatory drugs.

The second purpose is to establish the individual's level of absolute risk. A 65-year-old male patient who is a smoker, has a BP of 145/90 mmHg and who has already suffered a myocardial infarction (MI), will be at much higher risk than a 45-year-old lady with a higher BP of 160/110 mmHg and no other risk factors. Evidence of hypertensive target organ damage, such as LVH, proteinuria or severe retinopathy is of particular concern.

Absolute vs relative risk

Clinical Evidence defines the absolute risk as the probability (range 0–1) that an individual will

experience the specified outcome during a specified period. The relative risk is the number of times more likely (RR >1.0) or less likely (RR<1.0) that an event is likely to happen in one group compared to another. It is analogous to the odds ratio (OR) when events are rare, and is the ratio of the absolute risk for each group.

Investigations for all hypertensive patients

The basic investigations should include:

- blood biochemistry for urea and electrolytes, serum creatinine, fasting glucose and cholesterol
- urinalysis for blood, protein and glucose
- an ECG.

Urinalysis

Proteinuria and microscopic haematuria might result from renal arteriolar fibrinoid necrosis in patients with malignant hypertension. Such conditions can also occur in patients with non-malignant hypertension and hypertensive

Table 4.3
Secondary causes of hypertension

- Endocrine:
  - Cushing's syndrome
  - Conn's syndrome
  - phaeochromocytoma
  - hyper/hypothyroidism
  - acromegaly
  - hypercalcaemia
  - carcinoid
  - exogenous hormones, eg contraceptive pill, glucocorticoids
- Renal:
  - glomerulonephritis
  - diabetic nephropathy
  - polycystic kidney disease
  - renal artery stenosis
- Coarctation of the aorta
- Raised intracranial pressure
- Pregnancy-induced hypertension
- Alcohol and drug abuse
- Acute stress

nephrosclerosis. The risk of death is roughly doubled in those cases where proteinuria is present (for any given BP level). Glycosuria may indicate coincident diabetes mellitus.

Proteinuria and microscopic haematuria may also indicate:

- intrinsic renal disease
  - glomerulonephritis
  - polycystic kidney disease
  - pyelonephritis
- urological malignancy.

Haematology

Anaemia in a hypertensive patient may be due to renal impairment. Polycythaemia may be seen in patients with chronic obstructive airways disease, Cushing's syndrome, alcohol excess and very rarely, renal carcinoma. Plasma viscosity or erythrocyte sedimentation rate should be measured if there is a suspicion of some underlying vasculitic disease.

Biochemical investigations

Serum sodium concentration may be raised or in the high–normal range in patients with primary hyperaldosteronism (Conn's syndrome). In patients with secondary hyperaldosteronism, as occurs in chronic renal failure, serum sodium concentration can be low or low–normal. Low serum sodium levels are also produced by high doses of diuretics. Occasionally profound hyponatraemia may be encountered in combination therapy, such as Modiuretic (amiloride and hydrochlorthiazide).

Serum potassium concentration is usually low or low-normal in patients with Conn's syndrome, but the most common cause of hypokalaemia is diuretic therapy. Hyperkalaemia may be found in renal failure or with the use of some antihypertensive drugs such as the angiotensin-converting enzyme (ACE) inhibitors or the potassium-sparing diuretics (eg spironolactone or amiloride).

> Various serum sodium concentrations indicate different conditions, such as Conn's syndrome (high–normal concentration) or secondary hyperaldosteronism (low or low–normal concentration)

Life-threatening hyperkalaemia has been described in patients receiving an ACE inhibitor who then opted to consume a salt substitute (Lo-Salt), which contains potassium chloride instead of sodium chloride. ACE inhibitors and potassium-sparing diuretics should not be used together unless very careful monitoring of serum potassium is undertaken.

Serum urea and creatinine concentrations should be monitored as hypertension may cause renal impairment and some renal diseases cause hypertension. A graph plotting the reciprocal of the serum creatinine concentration against time may give an indication of the rate of deterioration of renal function, and hence predict the need for intervention and renal dialysis.

Primary hyperparathyroidism, which is associated with hypertension, causes a raised serum calcium concentration with a low serum phosphate concentration. As with serum potassium, these results may be affected by the use of diuretic therapy, which modestly raises serum calcium levels.

Hyperuricaemia is found in about 40% of hypertensive patients, in association with renal impairment. Serum uric acid levels rise with increased alcohol ingestion or the use of thiazide diuretics. Raised gamma-glutamyl transferase levels strongly suggest an excessive alcohol intake, assuming that other intrinsic liver diseases have been excluded.

Elevated serum cholesterol and triglyceride levels along with low high-density lipoprotein (HDL) cholesterol levels are synergistic risk factors that need to be assessed in all hypertensive patients and then treated if necessary. They may also be elevated very slightly by the use of some antihypertensive agents, such as the thiazide diuretics and non-selective beta-blockers.

> Two-fifths of hypertensive patients have hyperuricaemia in association with renal impairment

Electrocardiography

The ECG should be a routine investigation in all hypertensive patients, providing a baseline with which later changes may be compared. An ECG may show evidence of underlying ischaemic heart disease and is useful to screen for the presence of LVH. However, a normal ECG does not exclude the presence of LVH and there is a strong case for using echocardiography to more regularly diagnose cardiac enlargement.

For a given level of BP, if LVH is present, the likelihood of death from heart attack, heart failure and stroke is increased three- to four-fold. LVH is diagnosed on the ECG when the sum of the S wave in lead V1 and the R wave in leads V5 or V6 is ≥35 mm (the Sokolow and Lyon criteria). The presence of LVH provides:

- clear evidence of end organ damage
- a three- to four-fold increase in excess mortality
- an indication to the need for good BP control.

The prognosis is even worse if the 'strain' pattern of ST inversion is also seen in leads V5 and V6.

Investigations for selected patients

More detailed investigation is usually only necessary in a minority of patients (Table 4.4).

Twenty-four hour urine collection

The estimation of creatinine clearance is not necessary unless there is severe renal failure, but a 24-hour urine collection can provide valuable information in the investigation of hypertensive patients. For example, measuring 24-hour urinary sodium excretion may give

Table 4.4
Patients who require further investigations

- The young (aged <40 years)
- Those with severe hypertension (diastolic blood pressure >120 mmHg)
- Those with resistant or uncontrolled hypertension
- Those with a suspicion of underlying pathology, ie secondary hypertension

some indication of the patient's sodium intake and provide a basis for counselling. Cases of suspected Cushing's syndrome could be investigated with an assessment of the 24-hour urinary free cortisol. In those patients with a history suggestive of phaeochromocytoma, the 24-hour urine collection will allow measurement of catecholamines or their metabolites (metanephrines or vanillyl mandelic acid).

If urinalysis shows proteinuria, the 24-hour urine collection allows accurate quantification; those with more than 1 g proteinuria every 24 hours may require more specialized tests, including a renal biopsy.

> If more than 1 g proteinuria is seen over 24 hours in urinalysis, more specialized tests are required, including a renal biopsy

Imaging

A chest radiograph is not necessary for most hypertensive patients. Renal ultrasonography is useful in demonstrating unusual renal anatomy, such as:

- hydronephrosis
- abnormal polycystic kidneys
- diminished renal size.

A unilateral, smooth, small kidney may indicate renal artery stenosis. In patients with intrinsic renal disease the kidneys may appear 'bright' on ultrasonography. There are some important points to note if you are considering using a form of imaging (see Table 4.5).

Echocardiography provides the gold standard for the diagnosis of LVH

Plasma hormone concentrations

These are necessary to confirm the diagnosis of an endocrine cause of secondary hypertension. It is important that these tests are measured with the patient both fasting and supine, and then two hours later when the patient is ambulant.

Conn's syndrome results in a raised plasma aldosterone concentration with suppressed plasma renin activity. In contrast, secondary hyperaldosteronism gives rise to raised plasma aldosterone concentrations together with raised plasma renin activity. More recently there has been a trend to look for abnormalities in the renin:aldosterone ratio rather than simply high plasma aldosterone.

Table 4.5
Key issues to consider in imaging

- Intravenous urography is no longer used in the investigation of hypertension
- Renal angiography is the gold standard for the diagnosis of renal artery stenosis, although the procedure does carry some risk
- Magnetic resonance renal angiography has recently been introduced and this may become the investigation of choice to diagnose renal artery stenosis
- Computed tomography (CT) or magnetic resonance imaging (MRI) can be used for the localization of phaeochromocytomas or adrenal tumours causing aldosterone excess
- Standard renal radioisotope imaging now has little to offer in the investigation of hypertension
- Radioisotope imaging may also be useful in the localization of phaeochromocytomas using scans with meta-iodobenzylguanidene (MIBG scan)
- Iodo-cholesterol radioisotope imaging has little value in the diagnosis of aldosterone-secreting adrenal adenomas
- Echocardiography is primarily of use in the investigation of structural heart disease, including valvular heart disease and left ventricular dysfunction

---

Cushing's syndrome

Investigations for Cushing's syndrome should be conducted in all patients with a 'Cushingoid' appearance:

- a plethoric round face
- hirsute
- central obesity with red abdominal striae
- no obesity in the arms and legs.

Random cortisol assays can be misleading. An overnight dexamethasone (1 mg) suppression test is useful, although the differentiation between adrenocortical stimulating hormone (ACTH) secreting tumours and adrenal tumours secreting cortisol requires specialized endocrinological tests and computed tomography (CT) scans.

Acromegaly

Acromegaly may be suspected from the patient's face; it is investigated through glucose tolerance testing, measuring growth hormone levels and CT scans of the pituitary fossa. Primary hyperparathyroidism is diagnosed by the presence of a normal or raised parathyroid hormone concentration in the presence of a raised serum calcium concentration. The diagnosis of phaeochromocytoma is normally made from a combination of the patient's symptoms and the 24-hour urinary catecholamine analysis.

Blood pressure measurement

Despite the important decisions based upon it, BP measurement in clinical practice is fraught with inaccuracy. Variation in BP readings might occur because of:

- factors in the patient (biological variation)
- problems involving the observer (measurement variation).

Frequent observer retraining and a meticulous technique are vital. In an individual patient, BP can vary considerably. BP tends to be highest first thing in the morning and lowest at night, and is higher in cold weather and after consuming caffeine, tobacco or alcohol.

All adults should have BP measured routinely at least every five years until the age of 80 years. Those with high-normal values (135–139/85–89 mmHg) and those who have previously had high readings should have their BP re-measured annually. Seated BP recordings are generally sufficient, but standing BP should be measured in elderly or diabetic patients to exclude orthostatic hypotension.

> BP readings should be treated with some caution as a multiplicity of factors can skew the results

Coronary heart disease/cardiovascular disease risk

When assessing coronary heart disease (CHD)/cardiovascular disease (CVD) risk, it is best to use an average reading of several measurements taken at separate visits. This measurement is more accurate than readings taken at a single visit. In uncomplicated mild hypertension, the average of two readings per visit at monthly intervals over 4–6 months should be used to guide the decision to treat. In more severe hypertension, prolonged observation is not necessary or warranted before treatment. The average BP is only one factor determining cardiovascular risk in uncomplicated mild hypertension. Any formal estimation of CHD/CVD risk should also heed the consideration of age, sex, smoking habit, diabetes, total cholesterol:HDL-cholesterol ratio and family history.

Measurement devices

The most accurate device for a non-invasive BP measurement is a well-cared-for mercury manometer; however, mercury is likely to be outlawed in the near future due to safety concerns. Aneroid manometers are inaccurate unless regularly calibrated.

In the future, it is likely that most BP readings will be made with electronic oscillometric devices, although currently only

a few such machines have been carefully validated or certified for clinical use. For example, many devices have failed the British Hypertension Society (BHS) and/or the Association for the Advancement of Medical Instrumentation (AAMI) criteria, although the OMRON HEM 705 CP, OMRON M4 & UA-767 (A&D) have passed. Unfortunately, many devices are marketed without accuracy testing. O'Brien et al have published the full recommendations of the European Society of Hypertension on Blood pressure measuring devices.

> Testing equipment must be regularly calibrated to ensure the accuracy of BP measurements

Measurement technique

It is important that the correct sized cuff is used when measuring BP: the width of the air bladder should be about two-thirds of the distance from the axilla to the antecubital fossa, and it should encompass at least 80% of the upper arm. The use of too small a cuff will result in an overestimation of the BP.

The patient should be seated in a quiet room with the arm supported at the same level as the heart (Figure 4.1). The cuff should be inflated to about 20 mmHg above the systolic pressure as indicated by the disappearance of the radial pulse. It should then be deflated at 2–4 mmHg/second. The systolic pressure is recorded at the first appearance of the ausculatory sounds, while the diastolic pressure is indicated by the disappearance of the sounds, phase V.

Multiple measurements and monitoring

Blood pressure management decisions should be made on readings taken on several occasions over a period of time. Some individuals exhibit hypertension only in the presence of healthcare professionals, especially doctors. This 'white-coat' hypertension should be suspected in patients who:

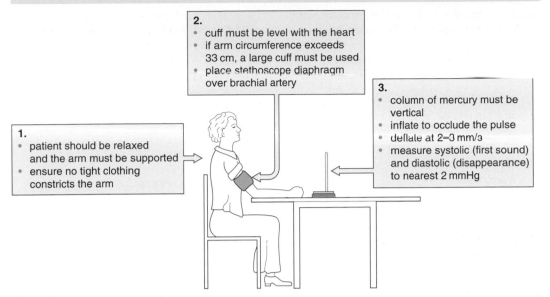

2.
- cuff must be level with the heart
- if arm circumference exceeds 33 cm, a large cuff must be used
- place stethoscope diaphragm over brachial artery

3.
- column of mercury must be vertical
- inflate to occlude the pulse
- deflate at 2–3 mm/s
- measure systolic (first sound) and diastolic (disappearance) to nearest 2 mmHg

1.
- patient should be relaxed and the arm must be supported
- ensure no tight clothing constricts the arm

Figure 4.1
Proper measurement of 'sitting' blood pressure.

- demonstrate persistently elevated BP yet have little or no evidence of end-organ damage
- who develop symptoms of hypotension on even small doses of antihypertensive drugs.

Home BP measurements with an automated device or 24-hour ambulatory BP monitoring (ABPM) will confirm the diagnosis of white-coat hypertension in these cases. ABPM also has a role in other special situations such as apparent drug resistance or hypotensive symptoms while on medication (see later). Normal home and ambulatory BPs tend to be slightly lower than clinic values. It should be remembered that almost all the data from which recommendations about BP management are made are based on surgery readings.

Systolic or diastolic BP?

In practice, systolic BP should be regarded as the more important. Both systolic and diastolic BP are highly correlated and outcome trials of antihypertensive treatment based on thresholds of diastolic or systolic BP have shown similar reductions in cardiovascular events.

Nevertheless, systolic BP is a better predictor of cardiovascular prognosis, irrespective of the underlying diastolic BP.

In the 1999 British Hypertension Society guidelines it is emphasized that treatment is recommended at a BP threshold of 140/90 mmHg; this means 140 mmHg systolic or 90 mmHg diastolic. Similarly, an optimal BP target of <140/85 mmHg means <140 mmHg systolic and <85 mmHg diastolic.

> Systolic BP is a better indicator of cardiovascular risk than diastolic BP

Ambulatory blood pressure monitoring

It is difficult to provide firm guidance on evidence for the use of ambulatory blood pressure monitoring (ABPM) to guide treatment, as all outcome trials in hypertension have been based on surgery or clinic BP, not ABPM. ABPM provides numerous measurements over a short time, and reduces variability and measurement error, when compared to the average of a limited number of clinic readings. Blood pressure readings taken by ABPM correlate more closely with evidence of target organ damage.

ABPM may be indicated in the following circumstances:

- when BP shows unusual variability
- in hypertension resistant to drug therapy, defined as BP >150/90 mmHg on a regimen of three or more antihypertensive drugs
- when symptoms suggest the possibility of hypotension
- to diagnose white-coat hypertension.

It is not necessary or feasible to perform ABPM to exclude 'white-coat' hypertension in all hypertensive patients. The term white-coat hypertension has been widely used to describe regular hypertension in the clinic with consistent normotension by ABPM. In these patients, there is a systematic 'clinic-to-ABPM' difference in the population that is related to the level of clinic BP. White-coat hypertension is considered to be present only when the 'clinic-to-ABPM' difference exceeds the average difference in the population. White-coat hypertension may not need treatment. These patients should be kept under observation as many do develop changes in endothelial function, intima-thickness, echocardiography etc that are intermediate between normotensive patients and overt hypertensive patients (Table 4.6).

| ABPM can be used to provide additional readings for BP, but not to exclude white-coat hypertension |

Thus, patients left untreated on the basis of ABPM will need to be followed up yearly, with reassessment of BP and cardiovascular risk. The annual reassessment may require repeated ABPM measurement.

When interpreting ABPM results, the average daytime BP should be used for treatment decisions, not the average BP over a full 24 hours. Any BP measured by ABPM is systematically lower than surgery measurements in hypertensive and normotensive people. Thus an ABPM average daytime BP of 148/83 mmHg is approximately equivalent to a surgery BP of 160/90 mmHg, and this may require treatment in some patients.

BP measurement at home

Evidence on the benefit of self-measurement of BP is less extensive than for ABPM, but many of the same considerations apply. Importantly, the 1999 British Hypertension Society guidelines recommend that measurements made at home need to be 'adjusted' upwards by approximately 12/7 mmHg (for equivalence to surgery or clinic measurements) when making treatment decisions.

Further reading

Ramsay L, Williams B, Johnston GD et al. Guidelines for management of hypertension: report of the third working party of the British Hypertension Society. J Hum Hypertens 1999; 13: 569–92.

The sixth report of the Joint National Committee on prevention, detection, evaluation and treatment of high blood pressure. Arch Intern Med 1997; 157: 2413–46.

1999 World Health Organization – International Society of Hypertension Guidelines for the Management of Hypertension. Guidelines Sub-committee. J Hypertens 1999; 17: 151–83.

O'Brien E, Waeber B, Parati G et al. Blood pressure measuring devices: recommendations of the European Society of Hypertension. BMJ 2001; 322: 531–6.

Table 4.6
White-coat hypertension as a cause of cardiovascular dysfuction

	Persistent hypertension	White-coat hypertension	Normotension
Isovolumic relaxation time	85*	87	70
E/A ratio	0.92*	1.01	1.21
LVMI	118*	86	99
Carotid stiffness	4.53*	4.32*	3.27

LVMI, left ventricular mass index. [Adapted from Glen et al. Lancet 1996; 348: 654–7]

5. Treatment

Starting antihypertensive therapy
Non-pharmacological management
Pharmacological management
Resistant hypertension
British Hypertension Society
guidelines

There is almost a dose–response relationship between increasing stroke and coronary risk with increasing blood pressure (BP). Conversely, strong evidence from randomized controlled trials suggests that a decrease in BP is associated with a marked reduction in hypertensive events. The question(s) posed with regard to hypertension management is no longer 'do we treat?', but instead, 'how to treat?' and 'who to treat?' (Figure 5.1). We need to identify populations at 'high risk' of hypertension, as well as the best way to manage these patients. Greater emphasis should be placed on BP targets and the choice of therapy administered.

When deciding on the most appropriate therapy, the modern approach is to take into account the patient's individual characteristics in terms of:

- concomitant disease
- risk factors
- social and economic considerations.

> Many factors must be taken into account when deciding on an appropriate treatment for a hypertensive patient

In the past decade, we have thankfully moved away from the rigid dogma of stepped care,

when all patients were started on a diuretic and then a beta-blocker was added if control was inadequate. It should be remembered that approximately 50% of all patients with hypertension will require more than one drug to control their BP, and one-third will require three or more drugs.

> Half of all patients with hypertension will need more than one drug to control their BP and one-third of patients will need three or more drugs

This chapter provides an overview of the management of hypertension, predominantly based upon the 1999 British Hypertension Society guidelines. There are many similarities with other guidelines, eg the Joint National Committee on Detection, Evaluation, and Treatment of High Blood Pressure (JNC–VI) and World Health Organization–International Society of Hypertension (WHO–ISH) guidelines.

Starting antihypertensive therapy

Absolute cardiovascular risk

In the 1999 British Hypertension Society guidelines, patients with cardiovascular complications (eg previous stroke or coronary disease) or target organ damage (eg left ventricular hypertrophy [LVH]) are recognized as having a cardiovascular risk that is sufficiently high enough to warrant treatment of even mild hypertension, for example 140/90 mmHg. For patients with 'mild' hypertension (average BP 140–159/90–99 mmHg) who were at variable risk due to other risk factors, the decision to start treatment is more difficult. Intuitive estimates of absolute risk are very inaccurate and while risk estimation is improved when additional risk factors are simply counted, it is significantly more accurate when all major risk factors are counted and weighted using risk functions derived from epidemiological studies, most commonly the Framingham risk equation.

> Even mild hypertension must be treated if the patient has additional cardiovascular problems

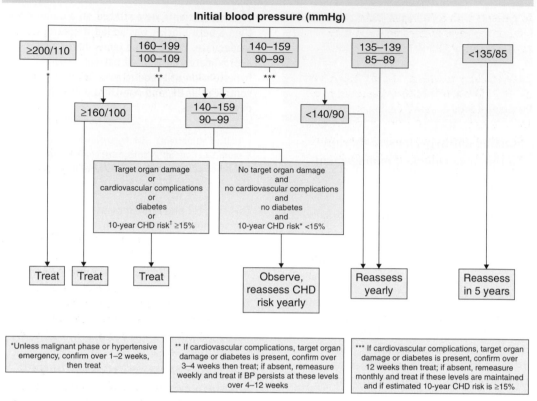

Initial blood pressure (mmHg)

*Unless malignant phase or hypertensive emergency, confirm over 1–2 weeks, then treat

** If cardiovascular complications, target organ damage or diabetes is present, confirm over 3–4 weeks then treat; if absent, remeasure weekly and treat if BP persists at these levels over 4–12 weeks

*** If cardiovascular complications, target organ damage or diabetes is present, confirm over 12 weeks then treat; if absent, remeasure monthly and treat if these levels are maintained and if estimated 10-year CHD risk is ≥15%

† Assessed with Cardiac Risk Assessor computer program or coronary heart disease risk chart

Figure 5.1
Blood pressure thresholds and drug treatment in hypertension [Adapted from British Hypertension Society. *J Hum Hypertens* 1999; **13**: 569–92.]

Assessing risk

The 1999 British Hypertension Society guidelines recommend the use of the Joint British Societies recommendations on preventing coronary heart diseases (CHD). The recommendations included:

- a computer program (the cardiac risk assessor)
- a CHD risk chart.

Both of these risk assessment tools are based on the Framingham risk equation. Either of these methods should be used to estimate the 10-year CHD risk to help rationalize treatment decisions. Alternatively, the 'coronary risk chart' issued by the Joint British Societies could be used (see inside front cover). The coronary risk chart is also based on the Framingham risk function and uses colour-coded bands to specify three levels of 10-year CHD risk: ≥30%, ≥15% and <15%.

The justification of this approach in the 1999 British Hypertension Society guidelines is that targeting antihypertensive treatment at absolute CHD/cardiovascular disease (CVD) risk is underpinned by evidence from meta-analyses of outcome trials. These show that the reduction in relative risk after antihypertensive treatment is approximately constant:

- 38% reduction in stroke
- 16% reduction in coronary events.

In patients with mild hypertension, treatment reduces cardiovascular complications by approximately 25%.

Treating patients with a 10-year CHD risk of ≥15% (CVD risk of ≥20%) corresponds to a 'number needed to treat' for five years of 40. This means treating 40 patients for five years will prevent one cardiovascular complication. Assessment of CHD/CVD risk also allows decisions to be made on the use of aspirin or statins in hypertensive patients.

At lower levels of CHD/CVD risk, BP management will be influenced by the patient's attitude to treatment and the benefit anticipated from treatment. It is recommended that all patients with an average BP of 140–159/90–99 mmHg should be offered drug treatment if:

- there is any complication of hypertension, target organ damage or diabetes
- the 10-year CHD risk is ≥15% (≈20% CVD risk) despite advice on non-pharmacological measures.

> Drug treatment in hypertensive patients can reduce the risk of strokes by 38% and coronary events by 16%

Monitoring

The 1999 British Hypertension Society guidelines recommend that when a decision is reached not to treat a patient with mild hypertension, it is essential to continue the observation and monitoring of their BP, at least once-yearly. Certainly, in about 10–15% of patients, BP levels rise in five years to levels clearly requiring treatment. Age is obviously an important consideration, and risk should be reassessed at yearly intervals. Non-pharmacological measures should be encouraged to lower BP and cardiovascular risk.

> Yearly monitoring of BP is essential, even in mild hypertensive subjects

Thresholds for intervention

When BP is seen to reach certain critical levels, therapy should be started as follows:

- Accelerated or malignant hypertension (papilloedema, fundal haemorrhages and exudates) or impending cardiovascular complications: admit for immediate treatment
- BP ≥220/120 mmHg: treat immediately
- BP 200–219/110–119 mmHg: confirm over 1–2 weeks, then treat
- BP 160–199/100–109 mmHg:
  - cardiovascular complications/target organ damage or diabetes (type I or II) present: confirm over 3–4 weeks, then treat
  - cardiovascular complications/target organ damage or diabetes (type I or II) absent: non-pharmacological advice, re-measure weekly and treat if BP persists at these levels over 4–12 weeks
- BP 140–159/90–99 mmHg:
  - cardiovascular complications/target organ damage or diabetes (type I or II) present: confirm and treat
  - cardiovascular complications/target organ damage or diabetes (type I or II) absent: non-pharmacological advice, re-measure at monthly intervals
- If mild hypertension persists, estimate 10-year CHD risk formally using the Joint British Societies 'cardiac risk assessor' computer program or the CHD risk chart. Treat if the estimated 10-year CHD risk >15% (≈20% CVD risk)

Non-pharmacological management

Before a patient is commenced on antihypertensive medication, it is always appropriate to attempt non-pharmacological measures to lower the BP. There are a few high-risk cases where they should be applied in parallel with drug treatment. Certainly, non-pharmacological measures can be synergistic with drugs, eg salt restriction and the use of diuretics. The elderly and

Afro-Caribbeans are examples where such an approach may be useful. Benefits of non-pharmacological methods are listed in Table 5.1.

> Non-pharmacological methods of lowering BP should nearly always be attempted before starting patients on antihypertensive drug therapy

A number of lifestyle modifications (eg weight reduction, salt and alcohol restriction and regular exercise) may produce significant falls in BP and can also improve other cardiovascular risk factors.

The epidemiologists would advocate that a population strategy could potentially prevent the rise in BP with age, reduce the prevalence of hypertension and the need for drug therapy, and reduce overall cardiovascular risk in a population. The public health initiatives for such a strategy include a diet that is:

- high in fruit and vegetables
- high in legumes and whole grains
- high in fat-free and low-fat dairy products, poultry, fish, shellfish and meat products
- high in all essential nutrients
- reduced in salt
- reduced in total fat, saturated fat and cholesterol
- low in alcohol (with no more than 2–3 units per day)
- calorie-controlled to prevent or correct obesity.

Table 5.1
Benefits of non-pharmacological methods to treat hypertension

- Lowers blood pressure as much as drug monotherapy
- Reduces the need for drug therapy
- Enhances the antihypertensive effect of drugs
- Reduces the need for multiple drug regimens
- Favourably influences overall cardiovascular risk

> In individual patients, changes in diet and lifestyle do lower BP and may also reduce cardiovascular risk

However, failure to adopt these measures may attenuate the response to antihypertensive drugs. Clear verbal and written advice should be provided for all hypertensive patients and also for those with high-normal BP or a strong family history.

The 1999 British Hypertension Society guidelines suggest that in patients with mild hypertension but no cardiovascular complications or target organ damage, the response to these measures should be observed during the initial 4–6 month period of evaluation. In patients with severe hypertension, non-pharmacological measures should also be instituted in parallel with drug treatment and should be backed up by simple written information. Effective implementation of these non-pharmacological measures requires enthusiasm, knowledge, patience and considerable time spent with patients and their family members. A summary of the non-pharmacological recommendations in the 1999 British Hypertension Society guidelines is as follows:

- Measures that lower BP
  - weight reduction
  - reduced salt intake
  - reduced alcohol consumption
  - physical exercise
  - increased fruit and vegetable consumption
  - reduced total fat and saturated fat intake
- Measures to reduce cardiovascular risk
  - stop smoking
  - replace saturated fat with polyunsaturated and monounsaturated fats
  - increase oily fish consumption
  - reduce total fat intake.

Weight reduction

Weight reduction results in BP reduction of about 2.5/1.5 mmHg for each kilogram lost and, in addition, could also improve lipid profile and insulin resistance.

> Every kilogram of weight lost results in a drop of 2.5/1.5 mmHg in the blood pressure

Salt reduction

Salt reduction from an average of 10 g to 5 g per day (5 g =1 teaspoon) can lower average BP by about 5/3 mmHg and is particularly effective in the elderly and those with higher initial BP levels. In most people eating a western diet, dietary sodium intake is grossly in excess of that required for good health. Hypertensive patients should be advised to avoid adding salt to cooking or at the dining table. Vast quantities of salt are contained in processed foods such as bread (one slice contains 0.5 g), some breakfast cereals and flavour enhancers such as stock cubes or manufactured sauces. These foodstuffs should be avoided. Salt substitutes containing potassium chloride may be beneficial, but can cause life threatening hyperkalaemia when combined with angiotensin-converting enzyme (ACE) inhibitors or potassium-sparing diuretics. Almost certainly, salt restriction can be useful in combination with antihypertensive therapy.

Alcohol consumption

Alcohol intake should generally be limited to <21 units per week. Hypertensive patients should be advised to limit their alcohol intake to 21 units per week for men and 14 units per week for women. Chronic excessive alcohol intake is associated with hypertension as well as other adverse cardiac effects, eg atrial fibrillation or alcoholic cardiomyopathy. Binge drinking is associated with an increased risk of stroke. Consumption of smaller amounts of alcohol, up to the recommended limit, may protect against CHD and should not be discouraged.

Regular exercise

Exercise on a regular basis should be encouraged, and the type of exercise should be regular and dynamic (eg brisk walking) rather than isometric (eg weight training). For example, three vigorous training sessions per week may be appropriate for fit younger patients, or brisk walking for 20 minutes each day for older patients. Indeed, 30–45 minutes of modest aerobic exercise, such as a brisk walk or a swim, three times a week would produce a modest fall in BP.

Fruit and vegetable consumption

Increased fruit and vegetable consumption, ideally two to seven portions daily, lowers BP in hypertensive patients by 7/3 mmHg. This effect may be a consequence of increased potassium intake. When this is done in combination with an increase in low-fat dairy products and a reduction of saturated and total fat, BP falls may be larger, averaging 11/6 mmHg in hypertensive patients and 4/2 mmHg in those with high-normal BP.

Cease smoking

Cigarette smoking substantially increases cardiovascular risk and is a greater threat than mild hypertension. Hypertensive patients who smoke should be given advice and help to stop smoking. The use of nicotine replacement therapies approximately doubles the smoking cessation rate.

> Cigarette smoking poses a greater cardiovascular risk than hypertension, but nicotine replacement therapy can double the smoking cessation rate

Saturated fat consumption

High serum cholesterol is additive to the risk of CVD. All patients should be advised to reduce saturated fat and cholesterol intake and to use polyunsaturated and monounsaturated fats instead. Most diet changes will only reduce serum cholesterol by an average of 6%, and there are great difficulties in implementing and sustaining these measures. Thus, many patients will need aspirin and statin treatment in addition to non-pharmacological measures.

Pharmacological management

It is now well established that hypertension confers an increased risk of heart attacks and strokes, and treatment of high BP reduces this risk. There is a wide variety of antihypertensive agents, although most can be divided up into the five major classes. Each of these drug classes has merits and disadvantages, as well as ancillary properties which all influence the choice for a particular patient. In addition, many patients require more than one agent to control their BP, so sensible combination therapy (with appropriate synergistic effects of the drugs) becomes important.

Choice of drug

With the wide variety of antihypertensive agents available, which is the ideal drug?

The cynic would argue that the ideal antihypertensive drug does not really exist. In assessing the drugs that are available, it is important to bear in mind those properties that would make an ideal drug for the control of hypertension. For each major class of antihypertensive drug there are indications and contraindications for use in specific patient groups (Table 5.2). When none of the special considerations apply, the least expensive drug with the most supportive trial evidence – a low dose of a thiazide diuretic – should be preferred.

> If a patient does not fall in to any of the special consideration groups, it is usual to prescribe a low dose of a thiazide diuretic. These drugs are inexpensive and have plenty of supportive trial evidence

Desirable properties

The ideal drug should have a predictable dose–response curve as well as an acceptable, recognized side-effect profile (Table 5.3). The issue of 24-hour control has also increasingly

been recognized as being important. Blood pressure tends to be highest first thing in the morning and this is when the majority of cardiac events occur. A short-acting drug, even if taken the evening before, may have worn off by the time the patient rises in the morning. A drug with a long half-life will still be protecting the patient after a night's sleep. A drug with a long half-life also has the advantage of only being taken once-daily which improves compliance, especially given that up to 30% of patients miss at least one dose each week. For example, the ACE inhibitor trandolapril maintains >50% of its activity 48 hours after the last dose.

As the purpose of treating hypertension is to reduce the incidence of hypertensive complications, particularly CHD and stroke, the ideal drug should have trial evidence to show that it achieves these ends as well as simply lowering BP.

> The ideal drug is a once-daily drug, giving 24-hour control, prolonging protection and reducing the risks associated when patients miss a dose

Drug studies

Recent long-term double-blind studies have compared the major classes of antihypertensive drugs (thiazides, beta-blockers, calcium antagonists, ACE inhibitors and alpha-blockers) and showed no consistent or important differences regarding antihypertensive efficacy, side-effects or quality of life. Overall, these outcome trials have shown significant reductions:

- 38% reduction in stroke
- 16% reduction in coronary events
- 21% reduction in cardiovascular mortality.

However, there were differences in the average response between drug classes that were linked to age and ethnic group. The reduction in coronary events observed in all trials was also less than the 20–25% reduction that is predicted from epidemiological observations.

Table 5.2

Compelling and possible indications and contraindications for the major classes of antihypertensive drugs

	Indication		Contraindication	
Class of drug	Compelling	Possible	Possible	Compelling
Alpha-blockers	Prostatism	Dyslipidaemia	Postural hypotension	Urinary incontinence
ACE inhibitors	Heart failure Left ventricular dysfuction Type I diabetic nephropathy	Chronic renal disease* Type II diabetic nephropathy	Renal impairment* Peripheral vascular disease†	Pregnancy
Angiotensin II receptor antagonists	Cough induced by ACE inhibitor‡	Heart failure Intolerance of other antihypertensive drugs	Peripheral vascular disease†	Pregnancy Renovascular disease
Beta-blockers	Myocardial infarction Angina	Heart failure§	Heart failure§ Dyslipidaemia Peripheral vascular disease	Asthma or chronic obstructive pulmonary disease Heart block
Calcium antagonists (dihydropyridine)	Isolated systolic hypertension in elderly patients	Angina Elderly patients	–	–
Calcium antagonists (rate limiting)	Angina	Myocardial infarction	Combination with beta-blockade	Heart block Heart failure
Thiazides	Elderly patients	–	Dyslipidaemia	Gout

*Angiotensin-converting enzyme (ACE) inhibitors may be beneficial in chronic renal failure but should be used with caution. Close supervision and specialist advice are needed when there is established and significant renal impairment
†Caution with ACE inhibitors and angiotensin II receptor antagonists in peripheral vascular disease because of association with renovascular disease
‡If ACE inhibitor indicated
§Beta-blockers may worsen heart failure, but in specialist hands may be used to treat heart failure
[Adapted from British Hypertension Society. *J Hum Hypertens* 1999; **13**: 569–92]

Table 5.3

Common or important side-effects seen with different classes of antihypertensive drugs

Common side effects	Diuretic	Beta-blockers	ACE inhibitor	Angiotensin receptor antagonist	Calcium antagonist	Alpha-blocker
Headache	–	–	–	–	+	–
Flushing	–	–	–	–	+	–
Dyspnoea	–	+	–	–	–	–
Lethargy	–	+	–	–	–	–
Impotence	+	+	–	–	–	–
Cough	–	–	+	–	–	–
Gout	+	–	–	–	–	–
Oedema	–	–	–	–	+	–
Postural hypotension	–	–	–	–	–	+
Cold hands and feet	–	+	–	–	–	–
Stress incontinence	–	–	–	–	–	+
Angioedema	–	–	+	+	–	–
Constipation	–	–	–	–	+	–

Few trials have compared different classes of drugs directly with regard to reduction in cardiovascular events and consistent differences between regimens based on different drug classes have also not been shown. The absolute benefit from treatment is smaller in women than men, but this is compatible with their lower cardiovascular risk.

Advocates of other drugs can point to reductions in surrogate markers, such as LVH or reduction of mircoproteinuria, to indicate their effectiveness. Large scale trials, such as ALLHAT (Antihypertensive and Lipid Lowering Heart Attack Trial) and ASCOT (Anglo-Scandinavian Outcomes Trial), which compare newer drugs such as calcium antagonists and ACE inhibitors with the well-established beta-blockers and diuretics, are currently in progress.

> Most major classes of antihypertensive drugs have similar characteristics such as efficiency and side-effects, although few trials have compared their effectiveness at reducing cardiovascular events

Thiazide diuretics

Thiazide diuretics act to reduce the reabsorption of sodium and chloride in the early part of the distal convoluted tubule of the kidney. This results in the delivery of increased amounts of sodium to the distal tubule where some of it is exchanged for potassium. The net result is increased excretion of sodium, potassium and water. Circulating volume is diminished, reducing preload on the heart and thereby lowering cardiac output and BP. With long-term therapy, autoregulation by the body's compensatory mechanisms results in vasodilatation, reduction of peripheral vascular resistance and return of the cardiac output to normal. Thiazides also have some direct vasodilatory properties. Thiazides are rapidly absorbed orally and produce a prolonged diuresis. Metolazone results in profound diuresis when used in combination with loop diuretics ('sequential nephron blockade') and therefore requires greater monitoring of patients.

The precise mechanism(s) of action of diuretics in hypertension is not fully understood. As mentioned, in the first few weeks of use, diuretics cause a fall in intravascular volume and total body sodium. Levels of circulating renin then increase and the intravascular volume and sodium levels return to normal; however, the anti-hypertensive effect remains. It may be that thiazide diuretics have a direct action on vascular smooth muscle. Newer thiazide-like agents, such as indapamide, may have an ancillary direct effect on the myocardium, resulting in regression of LVH.

> The best BP-lowering response is seen from low doses of thiazide diuretics, eg 12.5 mg hydrochlorothiazide or 1.25 mg bendrofluazide

There is no reason not to start treatment with a diuretic in the uncomplicated hypertensive and in fact many clinicians would loudly advocate their use. Whilst there is a flat dose–response curve in terms of blood pressure-lowering effect, the side-effect profile is significantly increased at higher doses and low doses should, therefore, be used.

Maximal response is obtained at relatively low doses, such as 12.5 mg hydrochlorothiazide or 1.25 mg bendrofluazide. Further increases in dose simply increase side-effects with little further effect on BP. Thus, higher doses of thiazide diuretics (bendrofluazide >2.5 mg or hydrochlorthiazide >25 mg daily) are unnecessary and should not be used. On the whole, standard doses of thiazides lower BP as much as other first-line antihypertensives. In some patient groups, eg Afro-Caribbeans and the elderly, thiazides are particularly effective. Conversely, they do tend to be less effective in younger Caucasian patients.

> Use of thiazides leads to increased excretion of sodium, potassium and water, and lowers cardiac output and BP

Thiazide trials

Thiazides are one of the classes of antihypertensives that have been extensively tested in large clinical trials. In early trials, thiazides reduced the incidence of stroke by the 40% expected from epidemiological studies, although the reduction in CHD was disappointing. This was perhaps due to the adverse metabolic effects of the large doses used. More recent trials using lower doses have demonstrated impressive reductions in both strokes and heart disease, especially in the elderly. At 28%, the reduction in coronary events in trials based on low-dose thiazides has been significantly larger than those in trials of regimens based on high-dose thiazides or beta-blockers. Low-dose thiazide-based regimens also significantly reduced mortality from cardiovascular and all other causes. The larger benefit on coronary events observed using low-dose thiazides is not necessarily related to the dose of thiazide as such. It may be related to:

- differences in age
- more effective potassium conservation in these trials
- chance.

In the LIVE study, the thiazide-like agent indapamide SR 1.5 mg was compared to enalapril 20 mg over a period of one year. Both agents significantly reduced BP, but only indapamide SR had a significant effect on left ventricular mass, reducing it by 5.8% compared to 1.9% with enalapril (Figure 5.2).

Choice of agent

There is little to choose between the various thiazides, although it seems prudent to use agents such as hydrochlorothiazide and bendrofluazide, which have been proven to be effective at low doses in clinical trials. Newer agents, such as indapamide, have fewer metabolic side-effects and, as mentioned above, may even regress hypertensive LVH on echocardiography.

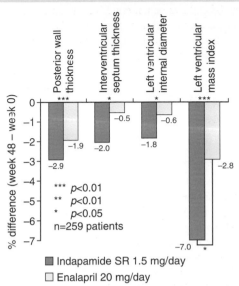

Figure 5.2
Beneficial effects of thiazides on cardiac dimensions; not only do they reduce the blood pressure, but they can also have a significant effect on left ventricular mass.
[Adapted from Gosse *et al. J Hypertens* 2000; **18**: 1465–75.]

Adverse effects

The main concerns about thiazide diuretics are the metabolic side-effects. At low doses these are less likely to be a problem. Predictably, thiazide diuretics cause hypokalaemia due to renal potassium wasting. Hypokalaemia may result in ventricular arrhythmias and cause adverse drug effects in patients on digoxin or drugs that prolong the QT interval on the ECG (for example Class I antiarrhythmics, tricyclic antidepressants antihistamines).

Acute gout is another common side-effect of thiazides even when they are taken in low doses. Hyperuricaemia can occur in about 30% of hypertensives, but is a poor predictor of acute gout.

Thiazides can increase serum LDL-cholesterol and triglyceride levels but this is much less of a problem with modern low doses. The diuretic-antihypertensive agent indapamide, given at a dose of 2.5 mg per day, seems to exert no relevant effect on serum lipoprotein compared to the thiazides. In hyperlipidaemic hypertensive patients, the benefits of reduction in cardiovascular risk from low-dose diuretics means these effects should not preclude their use. Indapamide may therefore be the drug of choice as it has the smallest effects on lipid metabolism.

There is also some evidence that diuretics impair glucose tolerance and increase insulin resistance, although the provocation of overt diabetes is rare. However, as mentioned previously, this effect is very small at the recommended low doses used in hypertension. Various trials have shown no detrimental effect in diabetic patients taking thiazides, with these patients deriving as much, if not slightly more, benefit than non-diabetic patients.

Rarer side-effects of the thiazide diuretics include:

- nausea
- headache
- rashes
- photosensitivity
- blood dyscrasias.

> Thiazides can cause metabolic side-effects but these are unlikely to pose a problem at low doses

Other diuretics

Loop diuretics act on the ascending limb of the loop of Henlé to inhibit the reabsorption of chloride, sodium and potassium. They produce a brisk but short-lived diuresis and are therefore unsuitable as first-line agents for hypertension as they lack 24-hour control. They do have a role in people with impaired renal function in whom thiazides are ineffective, and also in patients with hypertension resistant to multiple drug therapy who often have fluid overload. Furthermore, they may be synergistic with agents such as the ACE inhibitors.

Potassium-sparing diuretics, such as amiloride and triamterene, produce little reduction in BP. They may be useful in combination with other diuretics to prevent hypokalaemia. Spironolactone is a specific aldosterone antagonist with a particular role in primary hyperaldosteronism, also called Conn's syndrome, and recent evidence would support its use in patients with heart failure.

Beta-adrenergic receptor blockers

Beta-adrenergic receptor blockers (beta-blockers) act by blocking the action of noradrenaline at beta-adrenoreceptors throughout the circulatory system and elsewhere in the body. Their major effect is to slow the heart rate and reduce the force of contraction of the heart. Beta-blockers also cause some reduction in both renin release and central sympathetic tone.

Mode of action

The beta$_1$-receptor blockers or cardioselective agents, such as atenolol, have relatively less action on beta$_2$-adrenoreceptors in the bronchi and peripheral vessels, when compared to a non-selective agent like propranolol. This reduces (but does not totally abolish) beta$_2$-receptor mediated side-effects. The lipid soluble beta-blockers (eg propranolol and metoprolol) cross the blood–brain barrier more readily and are associated with a higher incidence of side-effects, including sleep disturbance and nightmares.

Some beta-blockers, such as pindolol, have intrinsic sympathomimetic activity. They stimulate beta-adrenoreceptors when the background sympathetic nervous activity is low and block beta-adrenoreceptors when background sympathetic nervous activity is high. They cause less bradycardia and fewer problems with cold extremities than conventional beta-blockers, but in practice are not regularly used in the treatment of hypertension.

Labetalol and carvedilol have both alpha-blocking and beta$_1$-blocking properties, leading to a reduction in peripheral vascular resistance as well as slowing the heart rate. They have the disadvantage of possessing the side-effects of both classes of drug. In addition to its beta$_1$-blocking properties, carvedilol also has antioxidant effects, which may reduce endothelial damage and lower levels of highly atherogenic oxidized LDL-cholesterol.

Efficacy

Beta-blockers are useful as first-line antihypertensive agents although they tend to be less effective in the elderly and in Afro-Caribbean patients. In these patients beta-blockers should not be used as monotherapy although this can be compensated for by using high doses or combination with a diuretic. When treating hypertension it is best to choose a beta-blocker with high relative cardioselectivity and low lipid solubility to reduce side-effects. Beta-blockers have also been shown to reduce the incidence of recurrent fatal and non-fatal myocardial infarction (MI) and sudden death in patients following a first MI. Beta-blockers are also useful if there is concomitant angina. Recent data supports the use of some beta-blockes in patients with heart failure due to left ventricular systolic impairment. These drugs include:

* carvedilol
* bisoprolol
* metoprolol.

Adverse effects and contraindications

Most of the side-effects of beta-blockers are predictable from their pharmacology. For example, beta-blockers slow the rate of conduction at the atrio-ventricular node and are thus contraindicated in patients with second and third degree heart block. Sinus bradycardia is common and is not a reason to stop beta-blockers unless the patient is symptomatic or the heart rate falls below 40 beats/min.

Small doses of beta-blockers can cause bronchospasm due to a blockade of the pulmonary beta$_2$-adrenoreceptors. This problem is less common with cardioselective agents; even so, all beta-blockers are contraindicated in asthma.

The blockade of beta-receptors in the peripheral circulation causes vasoconstriction, at least in the immediate term, and beta-blockers are therefore contraindicated in patients with rest ischaemia of the legs. Nevertheless, they are reasonably well tolerated in those with a lesser degree of peripheral vascular disease, especially if a cardioselective agent is used. Lipid soluble agents can cause central nervous system side-effects, eg insomnia, nightmares and fatigue. Exercise capacity may be reduced by the beta-blockers and patients may experience tiredness and fatigue. As with most pharmacologically treated patients, impotence has been reported.

> The side-effects of beta-blockers can usually be predicted, eg slowing the rate of conduction at the atrio-ventricular node

Diabetes

Like diuretics, non-selective beta-blockers can worsen glucose intolerance and hyperlipidaemia. In diabetics prone to hypoglycaemia, beta-blockers could theoretically reduce the awareness of low blood glucose. Nevertheless, many diabetic hypertensive patients have good reasons to be on a beta-blocker, such as a previous myocardial infarction or left ventricular systolic impairment, and should not be denied them because of concerns about the metabolic side-effects.

Beta-blockers may also promote weight gain and in the Captopril Prevention Project (CAPP), treatment based on beta-blockers and thiazides resulted in significantly more patients (approximately 21%) developing diabetes over five years when compared to treatment based on the ACE inhibitors. In the LIFE trial there was a reduced progression to diabetes in the losartan arm compared with atenolol. However, body weight and metabolic changes did not adversely influence the efficacy of antihypertensive therapy at reducing cardiovascular morbidity and mortality.

A study of 12,550 adults aged 45 to 64 years who did not have diabetes; subjects with hypertension who were taking thiazide diuretics were not at a greater risk of developing diabetes than subjects with hypertension who were not receiving any antihypertensive therapy. In contrast, hypertensive patients who were taking beta-blockers had a 28% higher risk of subsequent diabetes.

The concern about the risk of diabetes should not discourage physicians from prescribing thiazide diuretics to nondiabetic adults who have hypertension. The use of beta-blockers appears to (slightly) increase the risk of diabetes, but this potential adverse effect must be weighed against the proven benefits of beta-blockers in reducing the risk of cardiovascular events.

> In one study, 21% of patients treated with beta-blockers and thiazide diuretics went on to develop diabetes over five years

Calcium antagonists

Calcium antagonists, otherwise known as calcium channel blockers, act by interfering with the action of voltage-gated calcium channels in the cell membrane, thus reducing:

- the inflow of calcium
- smooth muscle contraction
- electrical conductivity.

Classes of calcium antagonist

In general, calcium antagonists may be divided into two classes:

- The dihydropyridines, such as nifedipine and amlodipine, act predominantly by causing peripheral vasodilatation.
- The non-dihydropyridines, such as verapamil and diltiazem, which additionally slow the heart rate and atrio-ventricular node conduction.

The older calcium antagonists, such as nifedipine, have short half-lives and may cause

rapid vasodilatation, a reflex tachycardia and catecholamine surges, which increase adverse effects and may aggravate myocardial ischaemia. Certainly, short-acting nifedipine capsules should not be used. The tendency to crush and give them sublingually is illogical, as they are not absorbed from the buccal mucosa. The crushed nifedipine capsule also alters the pharmacokinetics, which can cause erratic falls in BP. Longer acting agents such as amlodipine or slow release preparations of nifedipine partially overcome these problems.

> There are two classes of calcium antagonists: dihydropyridines (eg nifedipine and amlodipine) and non-dihydropyridines (eg verapamil and diltiazem)

Pharmacosurveillance case-control studies and trials

In the mid-1990s, a series of pharmacosurveillance case-control studies suggested that the short-acting dihydropyridine calcium antagonists (such as nifedipine capsules) actually increased the risk of:

- coronary events
- cancer
- bleeding
- depression
- suicide
- other adverse events.

There is little biological plausibility for some of the adverse effects proposed.

Recent data from the Syst-Eur trial demonstrated that antihypertensive treatment with the short-acting dihydropyridine calcium antagonist nitrendipine, convincingly reduced strokes and heart attacks, without an increase in conditions previously attributed to the calcium antagonists (eg tumours, bleeding and non-cardiac death). Recent trials (INSIGHT, NORDIL) show no significant difference between the calcium antagonists and 'conventional' antihypertensive drugs (diuretics, beta-blockers).

Pahor *et al* published a meta-analysis of 9 eligible trials that included 27,743 participants, and reported that the calcium antagonists and other drugs achieved similar control of both systolic and diastolic blood pressure. However compared with the 15,044 patients assigned either diuretics, beta-blockers, ACE inhibitors, or clonidine, the 12,699 people assigned calcium antagonists had a significantly higher risk of acute myocardial infarction (MI), congestive heart failure and major cardiovascular events. There was no difference for the outcomes of stroke and all-cause mortality.

In contrast, Staessen *et al* published a meta-analysis of 9 randomized trials comparing treatments in 62,605 hypertensive patients which suggested that calcium channel blockers provided more reduction in the risk of stroke and less reduction in the risk of MI.

Thus, blood pressure control is important and probably all antihypertensive drugs have similar long-term efficacy and safety. Calcium channel blockers might well be especially effective in stroke prevention. Overall, the evidence available strongly suggests that the benefits of dihydropyridine calcium antagonist treatment clearly exceed any risks. Verapamil and diltiazem may also be useful post-MI (in the absence of left ventricular dysfunction) and in controlling the ventricular rate in artial fibrillation.

Adverse effects

The main side-effect with calcium antagonists is ankle oedema due to vasodilatation which also causes headache, flushing and palpitation, especially with short-acting dihydropyridines. Some side-effects can be offset by combining a calcium antagonist with a beta-blocker.

Verapamil reduces intestinal motility and can cause significant constipation, but more seriously it can cause heart block, especially in those with underlying conduction problems. Verapamil should not be prescribed with a beta-blocker due to the risk of asystole, complete heart block or heart failure. Diltiazem

can similarly cause gastro-intestinal and conduction problems, although less frequently than verapamil. Verapamil, diltiazem and short-acting dihydropyridines are best avoided in patients with heart failure. Short acting nifedipine may be dangerous, but the long-acting dihydropyridines, such as amlodipine and felodipine, are neutral in heart failure and would be useful for the concomitant treatment of hypertension or angina in these patients.

> The main side-effect of calcium antagonists is ankle oedema, but this can sometimes be offset by combining with a beta-blocker (though not verapamil)

Alpha$_1$-adrenoreceptor blockers

The alpha$_1$-adrenoreceptor blockers (alpha-blockers) cause vasodilatation by blocking the action of noradrenaline at post-synaptic alpha$_1$-receptors in arteries and veins. This results in a fall in peripheral resistance without a compensatory rise in cardiac output. The older alpha$_1$-blocker, prazosin, is short acting and tends to produce precipitate falls in BP; the longer-acting doxazosin combines the advantage of a more gentle reduction in BP with once-daily dosing.

Alpha$_1$-adrenoreceptor blockers produce comparable reductions in BP to first-line antihypertensive drugs. They are useful as a third-line drug, producing good falls in BP where using two agents combined has failed. In contrast to the beta-blockers and diuretics, alpha$_1$-adrenoreceptor blockers modestly improve serum lipid and glucose tolerance, but whether or not this translates into improved outcomes is unknown, particularly with the lack of data on these agents.

> The alpha$_1$-adrenoreceptor blockers produce vasodilatation by blocking the action of noradrenaline in both arteries and veins, leading to a reduction in peripheral resistance without an increase in cardiac output to compensate

The ALLHAT trial

One worrying analysis from the ALLHAT trial on doxazosin has been highlighted. In January 2000, an independent review committee recommended termination of the doxazosin arm (n=9067) of ALLHAT on account of a 25% higher rate of combined CVD, a major secondary end-point of hypertension. After four years, 86% of patients assigned to chlorthalidone were still taking the drug as opposed to 75% in the doxazosin arm, and the mean systolic BP was 135 mmHg in the chlorthalidone group and 137 mmHg in the doxazosin group. Diastolic BPs were similar in the two arms of the trial.

For doxazosin versus chlorthalidone, the relative risk of developing:

- combined CVD endpoint = 1.25
- heart failure = 2.04
- stroke = 1.19.

Thus, it appeared that chlorthalidone, a cheaper drug, was superior to doxazosin for hypertension control, drug compliance and reduction of cardiovascular complications. For some drugs, BP reduction (identical in both arms in this trial) may be an inadequate marker of health benefits in hypertension. Also, antihypertensive drugs could have effects independent of BP lowering that may result in benefits to patients. The ALLHAT trial continues for other treatment arms.

Adverse effects

Alpha$_1$-adrenoreceptor blockers are, on the whole, well tolerated – the main side-effect being postural hypotension with the shorter acting agents. In women, alpha$_1$-adrenoreceptor blockers may cause urinary incontinence, and in men they may improve the symptoms of benign prostatic hypertrophy. Like most antihypertensive drugs, alpha$_1$-adrenoreceptor blockers can cause headache and fatigue.

Angiotensin-converting enzyme inhibitors

Angiotensin-converting enzyme (ACE) inhibitors have become increasingly popular over the past decade. They work by blocking the renin–angiotensin system, inhibiting the conversion of the inactive angiotensin I to the powerful vasoconstrictor and stimulator of aldosterone release, angiotensin II. This results in decreased peripheral vascular resistance and also a reduction in the levels of the sodium-retaining hormone aldosterone. ACE inhibitors also reduce the breakdown of the vasodilator bradykinin. This may enhance their action but is also responsible for their most troublesome side-effect of coughing. Furthermore, ACE inhibitors may improve endothelial function and reduce central adrenergic tone. They also have beneficial effects on renal haemodynamics, reducing intraglomerular hypertension and causing improvements in proteinuric renal disease.

> ACE inhibitors work by blocking the renin–angiotensin system thereby inhibiting the conversion of angiotensin I to angiotensin II

ACE inhibitors and the renin–angiotensin system

Because ACE inhibitors are competitive inhibitors of ACE, the secondary increase in levels of angiotensin I (due to loss of negative feedback) can overcome the ACE blockade. This leads to the return of angiotensin II levels to normal. It is also probable that there are other non-ACE pathways for the conversion of angiotensin I to angiotensin II, involving chymases and tissue plasminogen activator. For this reason ACE inhibitors do not comprehensively block the renin–angiotensin system.

ACE inhibitors as single agents

ACE inhibitors are effective as single agents in hypertension. There is generally little to chose between the large number of ACE inhibitors available. Recently, the CAPP study demonstrated that captopril was as effective as traditional antihypertensive agents (thiazides and beta-blockers) in preventing adverse outcomes in hypertension. Other ACE inhibitors, such as fosinopril, have the advantage of hepatic as well as renal excretion. Perindopril, lisinopril and trandolapril are agents with long half-lives and provide good 24-hour antihypertensive coverage.

Efficacy

The ACE inhibitors are particularly useful in diabetic hypertensive patients, where they slow the progression of diabetic nephropathy and are therefore reno-protective. Furthermore, these agents have been shown to improve diabetic retinopathy and possibly even diabetic neuropathy. ACE inhibitors are also used in patients with heart failure or left ventricular dysfunction, and this class is likely to be the most efficacious in LVH regression.

Recent evidence points towards an advantage of ACE inhibitors in cardiovascular prevention (ramipril in the HOPE study) and reducing mortality and morbidity in patients following stroke (perindopril in the PROGRESS study). For example, the ECG-LVH substudy from the HOPE trial compared baseline and end-of-study ECGs from 8281 patients at high cardiovascular risk who were randomized to ramipril or placebo and followed for 4.5 years in the main HOPE trial. In this analysis, ramipril prevented LVH or caused a gradual regression of LVH in 91.9% of patients; interestingly, 90.2% of patients assigned to placebo also had regression or prevention of LVH. Patients who experienced regression or prevention of LVH had a reduced risk of the predefined primary outcome (cardiovascular death, MI, stroke) and of congestive heart failure. Importantly, this effect was independent of hypertension or blood pressure reduction.

> ACE inhibitors may be most useful for treating patients with heart failure or LVH, as well as hypertensive patients who have diabetes

However, the ACE inhibitors tend to be less effective as antihypertensive agents in Afro-Caribbean patients and the elderly, due to their low renin state. This relative ineffectiveness can be overcome by using high doses or adding a diuretic. Nevertheless, in the African American Study of Kidney Disease and Hypertension, the trial had to be terminated early because the ACE inhibitor ramipril resulted in a significant delay in end-stage renal disease when compared with the calcium antagonist amlodipine.

Adverse effects

Although ACE inhibitors are successful drugs, they do have some disadvantages. ACE is not a specific enzyme and is involved in the breakdown of many other substances, such as bradykinin. The use of ACE inhibitors causes increased levels of bradykinin, resulting in the common side-effect of coughs and the less common complication of angioedema.

Coughs due to the inhibition of bradykinin breakdown are the most common side-effect of ACE inhibitors, occurring about five times more often than with placebo. Coughing is more common in women and older patients. The rare but more serious side-effect is angioedema, which occurs in 0.1–0.2% of patients, with a four-fold increase in Afro-Caribbean patients.

Serum urea and creatinine should be checked before and a few weeks after starting an ACE inhibitor as dramatic deteriorations in renal function can occur in patients with bilateral renal artery stenosis. Because of their effect of reducing aldosterone and thus potassium excretion, the ACE inhibitors can also cause hyperkalaemia. Rarer side effects of the ACE inhibitors include:

- rash
- taste disturbance
- blood dyscrasias
- vasculitis.

> Using ACE inhibitors can lead to increased levels of bradykinin, which has the side-effect of cough and the rare, but severe, complication of angioedema

First-dose effect

Significant first-dose hypotension is a fairly uncommon side-effect of ACE inhibitors, although large doses of short-acting captopril can cause sudden falls in BP. This first-dose effect is most common in those with volume depletion, such as in heart failure or in patients on large doses of diuretics. The limited data available suggest that perindopril is least likely to cause this initial hypotension.

Angiotensin II antagonists

These drugs act on the renin–angiotensin system; they block the action of angiotensin II at its peripheral receptors. Angiotensin II, an octapeptide derived from its inactive precursor, angiotensin I, by the action of ACE, is the final product of the renin–angiotensin system.

Angiotensin II is a significant contributor to the pathogenesis of:

- arterial disease
- hypertension
- LVH
- heart failure
- renal disease.

Whereas ACE inhibitors work by reducing the conversion of angiotensin I to angiotensin II, the angiotensin II antagonists block the action of angiotensin II at its peripheral receptors.

Mode of action

Angiotensin II antagonists have similar physiological effects to those of ACE inhibitors and produce similar falls in BP. As they do not inhibit the bradykinin breakdown, they do not cause coughing but may reduce the additional physiological benefits that bradykinin (a vasodilator) may bring. There is synergism of their antihypertensive effect by the addition of a thiazide diuretic. There is also some trial evidence that they may be useful in heart failure (eg valsartan in Val-HeFT, losartan in ELITE), left ventricular dysfunction post-MI (eg losartan in OPTIMAAL), regress LVH, improve proteinuria and improve diabetic nephropathy (eg losartan

in RENAAL, irbesartan in IDNT). As with the ACE inhibitors, they are somewhat less effective in patients who have low levels of renin, such as Afro-Carribeans and the elderly, but their action may be potentiated by the addition of a diuretic. Angiotensin II antagonists lower BP by decreasing peripheral vascular resistance without affecting heart rate and cardiac output.

There are currently six agents licensed in the UK, all of which are suitable for once-daily use:

- losartan
- irbesartan
- valsartan
- eprosartan
- telmesartan
- candesartan.

It appears that the angiotensin II antagonists may be an alternative to, or even offer further improvements over, ACE inhibitors in people with heart failure.

Adverse effects

The main advantage of the angiotensin II antagonists is their apparent lack of side-effects. One study comparing losartan with ACE inhibitors, beta-blockers and calcium channel blockers found that when using losartan, the incidence of any drug-related adverse experience (including cough) was similar to that of a placebo. First-dose hypotension occurred in only 0.4% of patients taking losartan 50 mg. Very rarely, angioedema has been reported with losartan. Like the ACE inhibitors, the angiotensin II antagonists may cause hyperkalaemia, renal impairment and hypotension but otherwise they are almost as well tolerated as placebo.

> Angiotensin II antagonists are well tolerated and very rarely cause any significant side-effects

Older antihypertensive agents

Older antihypertensive drugs still have a role in some special situations (eg pregnancy) and in resistant hypertension. Because they are cheap, they are popular in countries where hypertensive patients on low incomes have to pay for their own medication.

Central alpha-adrenoreceptor agonists

Centrally acting agents, such as clonidine and methyldopa, have previously been used to treat hypertension. These agents reduce sympathetic outflow by stimulating alpha$_2$-adrenoreceptors in the central nervous system. Although effective, they have been largely superseded by newer agents due to their side-effects of sedation and dry mouth, as well as the problem of rebound hypertension on withdrawal.

Mode of action and side-effects

These drugs (eg methyldopa and clonidine) stimulate central alpha$_2$-adrenoreceptors, resulting in a decrease in central sympathetic tone. This effect leads to a fall in both cardiac output and peripheral vascular resistance. Methyldopa is safe to use during pregnancy. Side-effects include sedation, a dry mouth and fluid retention. Furthermore, methyldopa can also cause autoimmune hepatic derangement and haemolytic anaemia.

New centrally acting drugs

Moxonidine represents the first of a new class of centrally acting antihypertensive drugs (the selective imidazoline receptor agonists) and is hoped to have the beneficial effects of centrally acting drugs without their side-effects. By stimulating central imidazoline receptors, moxonidine also reduces central sympathetic outflow without the dry mouth and sedation of central alpha$_2$-receptor blockade. Moxonidine also reduces peripheral vascular resistance without an increase in heart rate. The drug might also decrease plasma renin activity by direct action on the kidney and increase the excretion of sodium and water. Moxonidine has been shown to be superior to placebo and comparable to the main classes of antihypertensive drugs in lowering BP.

There are no long-term studies of these drugs with survival or cardiovascular events as end-points. One trial in heart failure (MOXCON) showed an increase in adverse effects with moxonidine compared to placebo, and was stopped early. In terms of side-effects, moxonidine causes fewer problems with dry mouth than clonidine, but other side-effects such as sedation, headache, nausea and sleep disturbance may occur. Overall, moxonidine appears to be as well tolerated as the main classes of antihypertensive drugs. Moxonidine also has no adverse effects on plasma lipids and glucose.

> Moxonidine stimulates the central imidazoline receptors and reduces central sympathetic outflow without the dry mouth and sedation side-effects of central alpha$_2$-receptor blockade. However, headache, nausea and interrupted sleep may occur

In summary, moxonidine is an effective antihypertensive agent. Although it is an improvement over clonidine it has not been demonstrated to have major advantages over more well-established drugs.

Direct vasodilators

The direct vasodilators, eg hydralazine, minoxidil, act directly to relax vascular smooth muscle, thereby reducing peripheral vascular resistance. The resulting activation of the sympathetic nervous system means that they can only successfully be used in combination with drugs that block sympathetic activity. However, the combination of hydralazine and nitrates may be better than ACE inhibitors for hypertensive Afro-Caribbean patients who develop heart failure.

Adrenergic neurone blockers

Such agents are now rarely used in the UK. Reserpine and guanethidine inhibit the release of noradrenaline from peripheral nerves, thus reducing:

- sympathetic tone
- peripheral vascular resistance
- cardiac output.

They cause postural hypotension and central nervous system depression. Where low costs are paramount, especially in the Third World, small doses of reserpine combined with a diuretic form an effective regimen.

Combined interventions to prevent cardiovascualr disease

In the context of overall risk, 'BP needs management' is perhaps the most important advance over the past few years. The importance of considering serum cholesterol levels, although obvious, has been much neglected. Indeed, hypertensive patients tend to have higher cholesterol levels than the general population and it is well recognized that those with both raised BP and raised cholesterol are at a particularly high risk of cardiovascular events. As long ago as 1987, it was found that only treating hypertension in patients with raised cholesterol had little impact on cardiovascular events.

The treatment of hypercholesterolaemia has been transformed by the introduction of the 3-hydroxy-3-methylgluteryl coenzyme A reductase inhibitors (also known as statins). The value of statins as primary prevention in high-risk patients has been clearly demonstrated. Two large trials (ALLHAT, ASCOT) on either side of the Atlantic are now underway to examine the value of statins in hypertensive patients with even modestly raised cholesterol levels. Recent data from the Heart Protection Study confirms the beneficial effect of statins in patients at high cardiovascular risk.

The anti-platelet agent aspirin has long been used in the treatment and secondary prevention of many of the complications of hypertension, but until recently little information has been available on its role in the management of the asymptomatic, hypertensive individual. Warfarin has also been found to be useful as a thromboprophylaxis in hypertensive patients with atrial fibrillation, but if BPs remain uncontrolled, such therapy carries significant risks, especially from intracranial haemorrhage.

Aspirin

Despite the strong pathophysiological and epidemiological associations between thrombosis and hypertension, there were little or no data on the routine use of antithrombotic therapy in hypertension, until the recent publication of the Hypertension Optimal Treatment (HOT) trial.

There are good reasons for treating hypertensive patients with antithrombotic therapy, especially when there have been previous heart attacks and strokes, ie secondary prevention. Examples include the use of aspirin following MI and cerebral infarction, and using warfarin if concomitant atrial fibrillation is present. There are no trials on the use of warfarin as a primary prevention in uncomplicated hypertensive patients.

HOT trial

The HOT trial was the first study to investigate the use of aspirin as a primary prevention in hypertension. In the trial, 75 mg of aspirin was given daily to treated hypertensive patients aged 50 years or above. This reduced cardiovascular events by 15% and MI by 36%, but had no effect on fatal events. This study showed the potential of aspirin to prevent 1.5 myocardial infarctions per 1000 hypertensive patients per year, which was in addition to the benefit achieved by lowering the BP.

The benefit seen in terms of reduced cardiovascular events was at the price of a higher incidence of bleeding events in the aspirin group. There was no increase in the number of fatal bleeding events (seven events in patients taking aspirin, compared to eight in the placebo group). However, there was a 1.8% increase of non-fatal major bleeding events

(129 events in patients taking aspirin, compared to 70 in the placebo group) and minor bleeds (156 and 87 respectively). These were mostly gastrointestinal and nasal. This increase in bleeding events was similar to that seen in other studies of aspirin (Figure 5.3).

> Aspirin can prevent up to 1.5 myocardial infarctions per 1000 hypertensive patients each year

Thrombosis prevention trial

In the thrombosis prevention trial of aspirin 75 mg daily for primary prevention, 26% of those studied had treated hypertension. The outcome was similar to that of the HOT trial:

- 16% reduction in all cardiovascular events
- 20% reduction in myocardial infarction
- no effect on fatal events.

In both trials, the number of clinically significant bleeding episodes caused by aspirin was similar to the number of cardiovascular events prevented by aspirin, suggesting that the margin between benefit and harm was narrow.

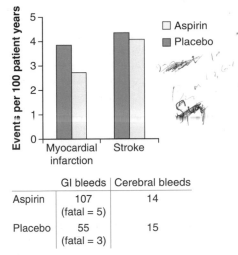

	GI bleeds	Cerebral bleeds
Aspirin	107 (fatal = 5)	14
Placebo	55 (fatal = 3)	15

Figure 5.3
Results from the HOT trial – showing that aspirin lowers the number of cerebral and gastrointestinal bleeds. GI, gastrointestinal.

It should also be noted that the HOT trial studied well-controlled hypertensive patients, and in the thrombosis prevention trial, aspirin was withheld when BP was above 170/100 mmHg. Furthermore, those who developed cerebral haemorrhage in the Thrombosis Prevention Trial had significantly higher systolic BP before the adverse event (158 mmHg versus 135 mmHg in those with no stroke).

Thus, hypertension must be well-controlled (BP <150/90 mmHg) before starting aspirin treatment for the primary prevention of CVD.

> It is important to have hypertension well controlled (BP <150/90 mmHg) before beginning aspirin treatment for cardiovascular disease

The British Hypertension Society guidelines state that 'aspirin 75 mg daily' is recommended for hypertensive patients who have:

- no contraindication to aspirin
- secondary prevention of cardiovascular complications
  - myocardial infarction
  - angina
  - non-haemorrhagic cerebrovascular disease
  - peripheral vascular disease
  - atherosclerotic renovascular disease
- primary prevention
  - BP controlled to <150/90 mmHg
  - age ≥50 years and target organ damage (eg LVH, renal impairment or proteinuria)
  - a 10-year CHD risk ≥15% when estimated formally by Joint British Societies computer program or risk chart
  - type II diabetes mellitus.

The 1999 British Hypertension Society guidelines make the point that patients with an estimated 10-year CHD risk of ≥15% will have their cardiovascular risk reduced by 25% using antihypertensive treatment. The addition of aspirin further reduces the risk of major cardiovascular events by 15%, giving a 'number needed to treat' for five years of about 90 for one cardiovascular complication and 60 for one myocardial infarction.

HMG CoA reductase inhibitors (statins)

Several primary and secondary prevention outcome trials have shown that statin treatment for primary and secondary prevention reduces major coronary events by 30%, reduces all-cause mortality significantly, and is safe, simple and well tolerated (see Table 5.4). Importantly, statin treatment substantially reduces the risk of stroke in patients who have CHD, which is an effect not seen in previous trials of lipid-lowering with non-statin drugs.

Statin treatment should therefore be targeted at a specified threshold of coronary risk and *not* at thresholds of lipid values. Statin treatment is theoretically justified at a 10-year CHD risk of 6%, but this would entail treating approximately 50% of all adults in Britain, and an even higher proportion of hypertensive patients.

Resistant hypertension

In view of new BP targets and the need for many drugs to achieve these lower BPs, many patients will be labelled by clinicians as having 'resistant' or 'refractory' hypertension. Careful examination would reveal that such a simplistic diagnosis may be fraught with problems.

A large data review from the USA (the National Health and Nutrition Examination Survey) has demonstrated that only 55% of hypertensive patients are being treated and only 29% have reached a target BP of 140/90 mmHg. Failure to achieve these goals can be attributed to several underlying causes, one of them being resistant hypertension. However, any debate about resistant hypertension is hampered by the lack of a generally approved definition.

One pragmatic definition for resistant hypertension is when a rational triple combination of antihypertensive drugs in appropriate doses fails to achieve adequate BP control (BP <140/90 mmHg).

The extent of this problem becomes clear when considering that up to 85% of patients referred to specialist hypertension clinics are reported to have 'resistant' hypertension when similar criteria to those above are used.

> Diagnosing resistant hypertension is made more difficult by the lack of a standard definition

Factors contributing to resistance

Several factors contribute to treatment resistance (Table 5.5). In primary care, truly resistant hypertension is most commonly caused by drug non-compliance. This is not an inconsequential problem as non-compliance rates of up to 50% have been

---

Table 5.4
Lipid-lowering therapy as primary prevention of hypertension

Study	Drug	Treated (CHD events/subjects)	Control (CHD events/subjects)	Odds ratio (95% CI)	Reduction (%)
LRC	Resin	155/1906	187/1900	0.81 (0.68–1.01)	19
HHS	Fibrate	56/2051	84/2030	0.56 (0.46–0.92)	44
WOSCOP	Statin	174/3302	248/3293	0.68 (0.56–0.83)	32
AFCAPS/Texcaps	Statin	56/3304	96/3301	0.58 (0.41–0.80)	42
All		441/10563	615/10524	0.70 (0.62–0.79)	30

Percentage reduction in CHD mortality = 29% and in all-cause mortality = 6%

CHD, coronary heart disease; LRC, Lipid Research Clinic; HHS, Helsinki Heart Study; WOSCOP, West of Scotland Coronary Prevention Study; AFCAPS/Texcaps, Airforce Coronary Prevention study/Texas Coronary Prevention Study.

Table 5.5
Causes of lack of response to therapy

- Non-adherence to therapy
  - instructions not clear and/or not given to patient in writing
  - inadequate or no patient education
  - lack of involvement of patient in treatment plan
  - cost of medication
  - side-effects of medication
  - organic brain syndrome (eg memory deficit)
  - inconvenient dosing
- Drug-related causes
  - dosage too low
  - inappropriate combinations (eg two centrally acting adrenergic inhibitors)
  - rapid inactivation (eg hydralazine)
  - drug interactions
  - nonsteroidal anti-inflammatory drugs
  - oral contraceptives
  - sympathomimetics
  - antidepressants
  - adrenal steroids
  - nasal decongestants
  - liquorice-containing substances (eg chewing tobacco)
  - cocaine or other illicit drugs
  - cyclosporine
  - erythropoietin
- Associated conditions
  - increasing obesity
  - alcohol intake >1 ounce/day of ethanol
- Secondary hypertension
  - renal insufficiency
  - renovascular hypertension
  - phaeochromocytoma
  - primary aldosteronism
- Volume overload
  - inadequate diuretic therapy
  - excessive sodium intake
  - fluid retention from reduction of blood pressure
  - progressive renal damage
- Pseudohypertension
- 'White-coat' effect

[Adapted from The sixth report of the Joint National Committee on Detection, Evaluation, and Treatment of High Blood Pressure (JNC VI), *Arch Intern Med* 1997; **157**: 2413–46]

reported with antihypertensive therapy. This is particularly a problem in younger patients who do not fully appreciate the need to treat what is usually an asymptomatic disease or risk factor. However, drug side-effects and multiple drug dosing need to be carefully excluded as possible reasons for non-compliance – simple measures such as a change in drug class and the use of once-daily dosing may help. Patient education and greater awareness of the risks associated with hypertension are also needed.

Other causes of resistant hypertension include concomitant medication, secondary hypertension, obesity, alcohol misuse and white-coat hypertension, which may be excluded by thorough clinical assessment and simple laboratory investigations.

Overall, the prevalence of secondary causes of hypertension amounts to about 5%, but investigations for rare underlying causes should be reserved for:

- patients whose initial assessment results are indicative of a secondary cause
- patients with an unusual clinical presentation (eg before the age of 20 years, after the age of 50 years, marked end-organ damage, BP >180/110 mmHg).

The patient's BP response to treatment can sometimes point to secondary causes; for example sudden development of renal failure or dramatic reduction in BP following treatment with an ACE inhibitor or angiotensin II receptor-blocker would be consistent with renal artery stenosis.

White-coat hypertension

White-coat hypertension should be suspected in patients who have resistant hypertension but no evidence of target organ damage. Some studies have suggested that up to 50% of patients referred to specialized clinics for assessment of their resistant hypertension had normotensive ambulatory BP readings. In hypertensive patients, there can also be a significant difference between office and ambulatory BP, the so-called 'white-coat effect'. If present, the readings in a clinical setting can exceed ambulatory readings by at least 20/10 mmHg.

Obesity, alcohol intake and cigarette smoking

A variety of other patient-related factors can contribute to resistant hypertension. Obesity is a 'pro-hypertensive' condition and weight loss of 10.4 kg reduces the mean arterial BP by 10/8 mmHg. There also seems to be a J-shaped relationship between alcohol and hypertension, where every unit of alcohol in excess of two units a day increases the BP by approximately 1 mmHg. Conversely, a reduction of alcohol intake in regular drinkers lowers BP by 4 mmHg. Another risk factor for resistant hypertension is cigarette smoking which causes a pressor response and thereby increases the BP.

Pseudohypertension

'Pseudohypertension' might be another underlying cause of resistant hypertension. In pseudohypertension, cuff sphygmomanometer BP readings are falsely elevated when compared to (normal) intra-arterial pressures. This condition is a manifestation of sclerosis of the brachial artery and is more common in the elderly. It should be suspected if the Osler's manoeuvre is positive, ie when a palpable radial pulse is present when the cuff is inflated above the systolic BP. However, the only reliable way of proving pseudohypertension is measurement of intra-arterial BP.

Concomitant medication

Concomitant medication is a frequently neglected cause of treatment-resistant hypertension. For example, chronic non-steroidal anti-inflammatory drug (NSAID) use increases the risk of developing hypertension and can impair the success rate of antihypertensive medication. NSAIDs can increase mean BP by about 4–5 mmHg. In addition to this hypertensive property, NSAIDs antagonize the effects of most antihypertensive drug classes. These effects are particularly important as NSAIDs are widely available without needing to be prescribed. Only careful history taking with direct questioning about NSAIDs can reveal this problem.

Practical considerations

A further important cause of resistant hypertension is a sub-optimal antihypertensive treatment regimen, which is even seen in tertiary referral centres. The choice of the first-line drug is very much influenced by the patient's age, ethnicity and coexisting disease(s), and initiation should follow or coincide with non-pharmacological methods, such as dietary advice, exercise and weight loss (Table 5.6).

Variable response to drug therapy

A variable response to the four major antihypertensive drug classes has been noted. In particular, age and ethnic influences on the renin–angiotensin system are of relevance. For example, patients aged <50 years are more likely to respond to ACE inhibitors and beta-blockers, whereas calcium channel blockers and thiazide diuretics are more effective in patients aged >50 years. These age-related differences can be explained by a different activation status of the renin–angiotensin system, with plasma renin levels declining with age.

Thus, blockade of the renin–angiotensin system with the ACE inhibitors, angiotensin II antagonists or beta-blockers tends to be more effective in young patients who are more likely to have high renin levels. In contrast, the diuretics and calcium channel blockers are good first-line agents in patients with low renin states, such as the elderly and Afro-Caribbeans.

Table 5.6

Strategies for resistant hypertension. Are they truly resistant? If no LVH, consider ABPM

- Simplify drug regime
- Check salt, weight, alcohol and exercise
- Check for NSAIDS, steroids etc
- Double check for underlying causes
- Remember effects of age and ethnicity
- Use powerful, logical combinations

ABPM, ambulatory blood pressure monitoring; LVH, left ventricular hypertrophy

Age and ethnic origin can influence the patient's response to drug therapy, particularly with drugs affecting the renin–angiotensin system

Concomitant factors

Concomitant disease states should also influence sensible prescribing (see Table 5.7). For example, patients with diabetes mellitus should receive ACE inhibitors because of the particularly favourable effects on nephropathy, retinopathy and LVH. Based upon the strength of evidence for reduction of cardiovascular mortality, a sensible choice as first-line drug therapy seems to be:

- a beta-blocker, angiotensin receptor blocker or ACE inhibitor in the young
- a thiazide diuretic or calcium channel blocker in the elderly or Afro-Caribbean
- an ACE inhibitor or angiotensin receptor blocker in the presence of concomitant heart failure
- a beta-blocker or calcium antagonist in patients with coronary artery disease
- an ACE inhibitor for diabetics.

Combination therapy

Many patients will not have their BP controlled by one drug alone. As most antihypertensive agents have fairly flat dose–response curves, using large doses of a single agent will produce significant increases in side-effects without much further lowering of the BP. The solution to these problems is to use a combination of two or more drugs. In general, 50% of hypertensives will require two drugs and one-third will require three or more drugs.

In the HOT study, fewer than one-third of hypertensive patients were controlled by monotherapy and more than one-third required a combination of three or more drugs to achieve optimal BP control. The major classes of drug generally have additive effects on BP when they are prescribed together, and most hypertensive people will require combinations of antihypertensive therapy to achieve optimal BP control. Submaximal doses of two drugs result in larger BP responses and fewer side-effects than maximal doses of a single drug.

Using drug combination therapy reduces the likelihood of developing side-effects associated with increasing doses of a single drug

Effective combination therapy will use drugs with different primary modes of action. Such combinations include:

- a diuretic with a beta-blocker
- a diuretic with an ACE inhibitor
- a beta-blocker with a calcium antagonist
- a calcium antagonist with an ACE inhibitor.

Beta-blockers, which lower cardiac output, can cause bradycardia and tend to increase peripheral vascular resistance. However, these adverse effects can be very successfully overcome when the drug is combined with a calcium antagonist, which causes vasodilatation and a reflex tachycardia. Diuretics can be synergistically combined with most other agents, except the calcium antagonists.

There is evidence that the combination of a non-dihydropyridine calcium antagonist and an ACE inhibitor reduces proteinuria more than either drug alone. The alpha-adrenoreceptor blockers can produce useful falls in BP when

Table 5.7
Useful antihypertensive agents in patients with concomitant conditions

Condition	Possible agents
Benign prostatic hypertrophy	Alpha-blockers
Hyperthyroidism	Beta-blockers
Migraine	Beta-blockers
Atrial fibrillation	Beta-blockers, verapamil, diltiazem
Osteoporosis	Diuretics

combined with most other antihypertensive agents. For third-line drug therapy, commonly used combinations are diuretic-ACE inhibitor-calcium antagonist or diuretic-beta-blocker-calcium antagonist. Fixed-dose combinations are not widely used in the UK. These combinations are convenient for patients and acceptable provided they are:

- used as second-line treatment when monotherapy is ineffective
- the individual drug components are appropriate
- there are no major cost implications.

> The most effective combination therapy uses drugs with different primary modes of action, so that the side-effects of one drug may be overcome by the action of another

Certain drugs should not be co-prescribed for the treatment of hypertension, eg:

- beta-blockers with verapamil
- potassium-sparing diuretic with an ACE inhibitor (although with careful monitoring and in the absence of renal impairment, spironolactone is used in heart failure).

The 'Birmingham Hypertension Square'

To assist in the rational selection of antihypertensive treatment, we have developed the Birmingham Hypertension Square for 'add-in' antihypertensive therapy (Figure 5.4). After choosing a logical first-line drug, the possible second-line agents are immediately adjacent, as indicated by the arrows. Third-line drugs can be chosen in a similar fashion.

The phenylalkylamine calcium channel blocker, verapamil, has not been incorporated into this concept and the combination of verapamil with a beta-blocker may even be dangerous. Instead, verapamil is a useful alternative to beta-blockers when the latter are contraindicated because of the side-effect profile or asthma. In one study, verapamil has even been shown to have synergistic effects in combination with the

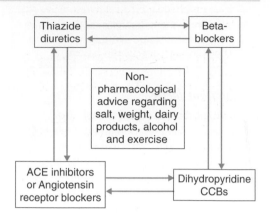

Figure 5.4
The Birmingham hypertension square. ACE, angiotensin-converting enzyme; CCB, calcium channel blocker.
[Adapted from Lip *et al. J Hum Hypertens* 1998; **12**: 761.]

dihydropyridine calcium channel blocker nitrendipine.

Due to sparse evidence, further 'add-on' therapy is subject to speculation. Alpha-receptor blockers or centrally acting agents such as moxonidine or methyldopa can be considered, but there are little data confirming their effectiveness and possible side-effects in combination therapy. Alpha-receptor blockers should perhaps be avoided as first-line therapy, particularly after the recent results of the ALLHAT study. The results suggest a higher risk of stroke and combined CVD endpoints (especially heart failure) in patients treated with doxazosin when compared to patients treated with chlorthalidone. Furthermore, the side-effect of stress incontinence limits the use of alpha-blockers in women. In resistant hypertension, the overall prognosis is more closely associated with the level of BP control rather than the initial severity.

British Hypertension Society guidelines

The guidelines set out by the British Hypertension Society are:

- Use non-pharmacological measures in all hypertensive and borderline hypertensive people.
- Initiate antihypertensive drug therapy in people with sustained systolic BP ≥160 mmHg or sustained diastolic BP ≥ 100 mmHg.
- Decide on treatment in people with sustained systolic BP between 140–159 mmHg or sustained diastolic BP between 90–99 mmHg according to the presence or absence of target organ damage, CVD or a 10-year CHD risk of ≥15% (according to the Joint British Societies CHD risk assessment program/risk chart).
- In people with diabetes mellitus, initiate antihypertensive drug therapy if systolic BP is sustained ≥140 mmHg or diastolic BP is sustained ≥90 mmHg.
- In non-diabetic hypertensive people, optimal BP treatment targets are systolic BP <140 mmHg and diastolic BP <85 mmHg.
- In diabetic hypertensive people, optimal BP targets are systolic BP <140 mmHg and diastolic BP <80 mmHg.
- In the absence of contraindications or compelling indications for other antihypertensive agents, low dose thiazide diuretics or beta-blockers are preferred as first-line therapy for the majority of hypertensive people. In the absence of compelling indications for beta-blockade, diuretics or long-acting dihydropyridine calcium antagonists are preferred in older subjects. For most hypertensive patients, a combination of antihypertensive drugs will be required to achieve the recommended targets for BP control.
- Other drugs that reduce cardiovascular risk must also be considered, including aspirin and statins.

[Adapted from *J Human Hypertens* 1999; **13**: 569–92]

Further reading
General

Felmeden DC, Lip GYH. Antihypertensive therapy and cancer risk. *Drug Saf* 2001; **24**: 727–39.

Felmeden DC, Lip GYH. Resistant hypertension and the Birmingham Hypertension Square. *Curr Hypertens Rep* 2001; **3**: 203–8.

Lip GYH, Beevers M, Beevers DG. The 'Birmingham Hypertension Square' for the optimum choice of add-in drugs in the management of resistant hypertension. *J Hum Hypertens* 1998; **12**: 761–3.

Lip GYH, Edmunds E, Beevers DG. Should patients with hypertension receive antithrombotic therapy? *J Intern Med* 2001; **249**: 205–14.

Ramsay LE, Williams B, Johnston GD et al. Guidelines for management of hypertension: report of the third working party of the British Hypertension Society. *J Hum Hypertens* 1999; **13**: 569–92.

Sever PS, Poulter NR. Hypertension drug trials: past, present, and future. *J Hum Hypertens* 2000; **14**: 729–38.

Thiazides

Beevers DG, Ferner RE. Why are thiazide diuretics declining in popularity? *J Hum Hypertens* 2001; **15**: 287–9.

Gosse P, Sheridan DJ, Zannad F et al. Regression of left ventricular hypertrophy in hypertensive patients treated with indapamide SR 1.5 mg versus enalapril 20 mg: the LIVE study. *J Hypertens* 2000; **18**: 1465–75.

Beta-blockers

Beevers DG. Beta-blockers for hypertension: time to call a halt. *J Hum Hypertens* 1998; **12**: 807–10.

Gress TW, Nieto FJ, Shahar E et al. Hypertension and antihypertensive therapy as risk factors for type 2 diabetes mellitus. *N Engl J Med* 2000; **342**: 905–12.

Messerli FH, Grossman E, Goldbourt U. Are beta-blockers efficacious as first-line therapy for hypertension in the elderly? A systematic review. *JAMA* 1998; **279**: 1903–7.

Calcium antagonists

Brown MJ, Palmer CR, Castaigne A et al. Morbidity and mortality in patients randomised to double-blind treatment with a long-acting calcium-channel blocker or diuretic in the International Nifedipine GITS study: Intervention as a Goal in Hypertension Treatment (INSIGHT). *Lancet* 2000; **356**: 366–72.

Hansson L, Hedner T, Lund-Johansen P et al. Randomised trial of effects of calcium antagonists compared with diuretics and beta-blockers on cardiovascular morbidity and mortality in hypertension: the Nordic Diltiazem (NORDIL) study. *Lancet* 2000; **356**: 359–65.

Hansson L, Zanchetti A, Carruthers SG et al. Effects of intensive blood-pressure lowering and low-dose aspirin in patients with hypertension: principal results of the Hypertension Optimal Treatment (HOT) randomised trial. HOT Study Group. *Lancet* 1998; **351**: 1755–62.

Pahor M, Psaty BM, Alderman MH *et al*. Health outcomes associated with calcium antagonists compared with other first-line antihypertensive therapies: a meta-analysis of randomised controlled trials. *Lancet* 2000; **356**: 1949–54.

Staessen JA, Fagard R, Thijs L *et al*. Randomised double-blind comparison of placebo and active treatment for older patients with isolated systolic hypertension. The Systolic Hypertension in Europe (SYST-EUR) Trial Investigators. *Lancet* 1997; **350**: 754–64.

Alpha blockers

Beevers DG, Lip GYH. Do alpha blockers cause heart failure and stroke? Observations from ALLHAT. *J Hum Hypertens* 2000; **14**: 287–9.

Major cardiovascular events in hypertensive patients randomized to doxazosin vs chlorthalidone: the antihypertensive and lipid-lowering treatment to prevent heart attack trial (ALLHAT). ALLHAT Collaborative Research Group. *JAMA* 2000; **283**: 1967–75.

ACE inhibitors

African American Study of Kidney Disease and Hypertension (AASK) Study Group. The effect of ramipril vs amlodipine on renal outcomes in hypertensive nephrosclerosis; a randomized controlled trial. *JAMA* 2001; **285**: 2719–28.

Hansson L, Lindholm LH, Niskanen L *et al*. Effect of angiotensin-converting-enzyme inhibition compared with conventional therapy on cardiovascular morbidity and mortality in hypertension: the Captopril Prevention Project (CAPPP) randomised trial. *Lancet* 1999; **353**: 611–16.

Mathew J, Sleight P, Lonn E *et al*. Reduction of cardiovascular risk by regression of electrocardiographic markers of left ventricular hypertrophy by the angiotensin-converting enzyme inhibitor ramipril. *Circulation* 2001; **104**: 1615–21.

PROGRESS Collaborative Group. Randomised trial of a perindopril-based blood-pressure-lowering regimen among 6,105 individuals with previous stroke or transient ischaemic attack. *Lancet* 2001; **358**: 1033–41.

Yusuf S, Sleight P, Pogue J *et al*. Effects of an angiotensin-converting-enzyme inhibitor, ramipril, on cardiovascular events in high-risk patients. The Heart Outcomes Prevention Evaluation Study Investigators. *N Engl J Med* 2000; **342**: 145–53.

Angiotensin receptor antagonists

Brenner BM, Cooper ME, de Zeeuw D *et al*. Effects of losartan on renal and cardiovascular outcomes in patients with type 2 diabetes and nephropathy. N Engl J Med 2001; **345**: 861-9.

Dahlof B, Devereux RB, Kjeldsen SE *et al*. Cardiovascular morbidity and mortality in the Losartan Intervention For Endpoint reduction in hypertension study (LIFE): a randomised trial against atenolol. *Lancet* 2002; **359**: 995–1003.

Lewis EJ, Hunsicker LG, Clarke WR *et al*. Renoprotective effect of the angiotensin-receptor antagonist irbesartan in patients with nephropathy due to type 2 diabetes. *N Engl J Med* 2001; **345**: 851–60.

Lindholm LH, Ibsen H, Dahlof B *et al*. Cardiovascular morbidity and mortality in patients with diabetes in the Losartan Intervention For Endpoint reduction in hypertension study (LIFE): a randomised trial against atenolol. *Lancet* 2002; **359**: 1004–10.

Parving HH, Lehnert H, Brochner-Mortensen J *et al*. Effect of irbesartan on the development of diabetic nephropathy in patients with type 2 diabetes. *N Engl J Med* 2001; **345**: 870–8.

Pitt B, Poole-Wilson PA, Segal R *et al*. The effect of losartan compared with captopril on mortality in patients with symptomatic heart failure: randomised trial – the Losartan Heart Failure Survival Study ELITE II. *Lancet* 2000; **355**: 1582–7.

6. Special patient groups

Diabetes
Coronary artery disease
Cardiac failure
Hypertension following a stroke
The elderly
Renal disease
Peripheral vascular disease
Ethnic groups
Hyperlipidaemia
Oral contraceptives
Hormone replacement therapy
Anaesthesia and surgery
Children

Many patients with hypertension fall into a number of special groups where there are either compelling indications against a particular agent from randomized controlled trials, or good reasons to believe that a specific agent will have favourable effects on a co-morbid condition. These 'special patient groups' are discussed here.

Diabetes

Hypertension and diabetes are a bad combination. Both risk factors significantly increase the risk of vascular mortality and morbidity, especially in association with other risk factors such as hyperlipidaemia or smoking (Figure 6.1). Hypertension is present in about 20% of patients with insulin-dependent diabetes and between 30–50% of patients with non insulin-dependent diabetes. This proportion (especially non insulin-dependent or type II diabetes) may be higher (approximately two-thirds) in patients of Afro-Caribbean or Indo-Asian origin (Figure 6.2).

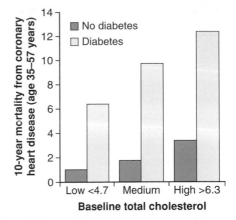

Figure 6.1
Diabetes, lipids and risk. [Adapted from *Lancet* 2000; **356**: 147–52.]

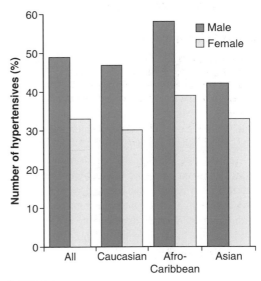

Figure 6.2
Cases of hypertension (BP >160/90 mmHg) in a diabetic clinic. [Adapted from Pacy *et al. Postgrad Med J* 1983; **59**: 637–90.]

Patients with diabetes suffer from:

● macrovascular complications (eg myocardial infarction and peripheral vascular disease)

● microvascular disease (eg diabetic nephropathy and retinopathy)

● an increased risk of heart failure and atrial fibrillation.

> Diabetes and hypertension combine to significantly increase the risk of vascular mortality and morbidity

In type I diabetes, there is clear evidence that angiotensin-converting enzyme (ACE) inhibitors reduce the progression of retinopathy, nephropathy and possibly even neuropathy – these drugs should be regarded as first-line agent in patients with these complications.

In type II diabetes, lower blood pressure (BP) targets (BP <130/80 mmHg) improve prognosis. Furthermore, reductions in proteinuria with the ACE inhibitors, calcium antagonists and, more recently, alpha-blockers have been noted.

Low-dose diuretics have also been found to be just as effective in diabetic as non-diabetic patients. Traditionally, drugs such as the thiazide diuretics have had the potential to exacerbate glucose intolerance and lipid abnormalities, although these metabolic effects are minimal at low doses. However, newer diuretics, such as indapamide, have been acknowledged as being more metabolically neutral. The ACE inhibitors (or failing that, the angiotensin receptor antagonists) are probably the first choice for patients with type II diabetes and proteinuria. They have the advantage of reducing the progression of diabetic nephropathy or retinopathy. The angiotensin receptor blockers are an alternative to the ACE inhibitors and may reduce the incidence of new onset diabetes when compared with beta-blockers. The calcium antagonists, beta-blockers and low-dose diuretics are also suitable in uncomplicated type II diabetes. The beta-blockers are generally safe, but non-cardioselective agents may blunt the hypoglycaemic response to insulin. The aim is to achieve not just 'good', but 'excellent' BP control.

Type I diabetes

In type I disease, an increased prevalence of hypertension is only seen in those patients with nephropathy (microalbuminuria or proteinuria), otherwise prevalence is similar to a non-diabetic population. In patients without nephropathy, the threshold for intervention with antihypertensive therapy is a systolic BP ≥140/90 mmHg and an optimal BP target of <140/80 mmHg (<130/80 mmHg in the WHO/ISH guidelines).

In patients with diabetic nephropathy, developing hypertension may indicate the presence of the nephropathy. Certainly, BP reduction and treatment with ACE inhibitors and angiotensin II receptor antagonists slows the rate of renal function decline in overt diabetic nephropathy. Treatment also delays the progression from the microalbuminuric phase to overt nephropathy. These drugs might have a specific renoprotective action in patients with incipient or overt nephropathy and are to be recommended as first-line therapy. For renoprotection, BP control is crucial and recommended BP targets should be achieved by multiple drug therapy.

> The first choice of antihypertensive drug for patients with type I diabetes is either an ACE inhibitor or an angiotensin receptor antagonist

The threshold for antihypertensive treatment in type 1 diabetes with nephropathy is BP ≥140/90 mmHg, aiming for a target BP <130/80 mmHg, or even lower (BP <125/75 mmHg) if there is ≥1 g proteinuria every 24 hours. If persistent microalbuminuria or proteinuria is present but BP is normal, these patients may still benefit from ACE inhibitors or angiotensin receptor antagonists. As is evident from the recent HOPE trial, the beneficial effects of ACE inhibition (ramipril in the HOPE Trial) are independent of the degree of BP reduction. In view of the high cardiovascular risk, statin therapy should be considered if a patient's total cholesterol is ≥5 mmol/L. Aspirin therapy may be used in type I diabetics with nephropathy.

Type II diabetes

Hypertension is very common in type II diabetes and patients that suffer from both conditions are frequently obese. In type II diabetes, hypertension is prevalent in over 70% of patients and may even precede the onset of diabetes. The presence of hypertension in type II diabetes is highly predictive of cardiovascular and microvascular complications with an overall 10-year cardiovascular risk of >30%. These are predominantly coronary events.

> The presence of hypertension in patients with type II diabetes increases the risk of microvascular and cardiovascular complications

Hypertension studies in diabetics

The threshold for intervention with antihypertensive therapy is BP ≥140/90 mmHg in type II diabetes. In the UKPDS (United Kingdom Prospective Diabetes Study) study, antihypertensive therapy was more effective in protecting against microvascular and macrovascular disease than tight glycaemic control. It was the only intervention that actually decreased mortality rates in patients with type II diabetes.

In UKPDS, patients with hypertension and type II diabetes assigned captopril or atenolol to achieve tight control of blood pressure achieved a significant reduction in risk of 24% for any end points related to diabetes and 37% risk reduction for microvascular disease. In comparison, intensive blood glucose control in the UKPDS decreased the risk of any diabetes related end point by 12% (p=0.029) and microvascular disease by 25% (p=0.0099). Diabetics from the Hypertension Optimal Trial (HOT) and the elderly diabetics with isolated systolic hypertension from the SystEur trial also showed marked benefits after receiving treatment, with a BP target <140/80 mmHg. Specifically, diabetic patients in the group with a target diastolic pressure <80 mmHg in the HOT study had a 51% reduction in major cardiovascular events compared to the group with a target diastolic pressure of <90.

In the Irbesartan Diabetic Nephropathy Trial (IDNT), the angiotensin II receptor antagonist

irbesartan was compared with amlodipine and with placebo in diabetic patients with overt proteinuria. Both drugs reduced the blood pressure by roughly equal amounts but only irbesartan caused any delay in the progression of diabetic nephropathy.

In the IRbesartan MicroAlbuminuria Type 2 Diabetes Mellitus in Hypertensive patients (IRMA 2) study, two different dose levels of irbesartan (150 and 300 mg daily) were compared with placebo in diabetic patients who had microproteinuria. This trial was able to demonstrate a statistically significant dose–response curve with the 300 mg dose of irbesartan being more effective than the 150 mg dose at reducing microproteinuria or normalizing albumen excretion.

In the Reduction of Endpoints in Non-Insulin Dependent Diabetes Mellitus with the Angiotensin II Antagonist Losartan (RENAAL) trial, losartan was compared with placebo in patients with overt diabetic nephropathy. This trial was able to demonstrate a 16% reduction in the doubling of serum creatinine and a 28% reduction in end-stage renal disease. Another finding which was considered as a secondary end-point was a 32% reduction in hospitalization for heart failure.

Suggested drug treatment

The choice of first-line drug favours the ACE inhibitors, with additional use for dihydropyridine calcium antagonists, low-dose thiazide diuretics and beta-blockers to achieve target blood pressures. The UKPDS study suggested that regimens based on ACE-inhibition (captopril) and beta-blockade (atenolol) were equally effective at reducing macrovascular complications, but the treatment groups were too small to be conclusive.

In type II diabetic subjects with nephropathy, hypertension accelerates the decline of renal function. This is slowed by treatment with antihypertensive therapy. While the ACE inhibitors (and more recently the angiotensin II receptor antagonists) have an antiproteinuric action and delay the progression from microalbuminuria to overt nephropathy, it is less clear whether or not they have a specific renoprotective action beyond BP reduction in overt nephropathy complicating type II diabetes. Aspirin should also be offered to all patients with diabetes and hypertension, as well as statin therapy for primary prevention, because their estimated 10-year coronary heart disease (CHD) risk is likely to be ≥30%.

Coronary artery disease

Hypertension is a risk factor for the development of atheromatous coronary artery disease (CAD). Nevertheless, many patients with angina and hypertension have normal coronary arteries on angiography despite having highly abnormal 12-lead resting ECGs with gross left ventricular hypertrophy (LVH) and strain, making the diagnosis of infarction or ischaemia difficult.

> Some patients with angina and hypertension may have normal coronary arteries on angiography despite having abnormal ECGs and severe LVH. This can complicate the diagnosis of ischaemia or infarction

Clinical signs

Coronary artery disease, as manifest by angina and myocardial infarction, is more common in patients with hypertension. There appears to be an almost dose–response relationship between coronary risk and increasing BP. While angina usually results from coronary artery atherosclerosis, it can also result from relative ischaemia in severe LVH. In any case, hypertensive patients with overt coronary artery disease are at particularly high risk of further cardiac events. In the peri-infarction state, BP may have fallen so that the diagnosis of hypertension may be missed and may only become apparent at subsequent outpatient clinic visits.

Suggested drug treatment

Effective treatment of hypertension may improve the symptoms of angina regardless of the drugs used. As beta-blockers are useful for secondary prevention after myocardial infarction (MI), they are the first-choice drugs for hypertensive patients who have sustained a myocardial infarct. If beta-blockers are contraindicated, calcium antagonists (eg verapamil or diltiazem) may be beneficial provided there is no evidence of heart failure or left ventricular dysfunction. Verapamil should not be given with a beta-blocker as it can result in:

- asytole
- heart block
- cardiac failure.

> Beta-blockers are the first choice drug to treat angina symptoms in hypertensive patients

There is some evidence that diltiazem may be beneficial following non-Q-wave MI. The dihydropyridine calcium antagonists (particularly nifedipine) should be avoided both in the immediate post-infarction period and in unstable angina. The presence of heart failure or left ventricular dysfunction post-MI is a strong indicator that an ACE inhibitor should be deployed. An angiotensin receptor blocker would be an alternative to ACE inhibitors.

Patients taking thiazide diuretics who are admitted with MI should have their serum potassium concentrations checked; they may have hypokalaemia, which can exacerbate the tendency to cardiac arrhythmia and sudden death.

Cardiac failure

Usually heart failure develops in the hypertensive patient in association with CAD. Rarely, severe hypertension can be associated with heart failure. Echocardiography can help diagnose structural heart disease and assess cardiac function.

Suggested drug treatment

There are few data available about the best drug for those with both hypertension and heart failure. Caution is needed when using verapamil or diltiazem for hypertension in patients with heart failure. Many trials have firmly established the role of ACE inhibitors in patients with heart failure (Figure 6.3), and the benefits are greater if the heart failure is more severe – many such patients have co-existing hypertension.

Recent data point to the angiotensin II receptor antagonists as an alternative to the ACE inhibitors. One study (Val-HeFT – the valsartan heart failure trial) suggested that adding valsartan to an ACE inhibitor has a beneficial effect in reducing hospitalizations, although not in patients already taking a beta-blocker. However, more data are required before the addition of an ACE inhibitor to an angiotensin II receptor antagonist becomes routine clinical practice. Most patients with heart failure will also require a diuretic and combining an ACE inhibitor (or angiotensin II receptor antagonist) and a diuretic may be sufficient to control BP.

The combination of hydralazine and nitrates is used if ACE inhibitors are contraindicated or cause side-effects, although this regime may be better than ACE inhibitors for Afro-Caribbean hypertension patients with heart failure.

Beta-blockers

In stable patients with chronic heart failure, a beta-blocker (eg carvedilol, bisoprolol or metoprolol) added to an ACE inhibitor and a diuretic has a beneficial effect on mortality and morbidity. Beta-blockers should be initiated in patients with heart failure under specialist advice and should be started at a low-dose and uptitrated slowly. Additional blockade of the renin–angiotensin–aldosterone system, using the aldosterone antagonist spironolactone, also significantly reduces mortality and morbidity in patients established on standard therapy (including the ACE inhibitors), see Figure 6.4.

> In hypertensive patients with heart failure, beta-blockers should be started at a low dose and uptitrated gradually

Hypertension following a stroke

Uncontrolled hypertension in association with cerebrovascular disease is a risk factor for further cerebrovascular events. It is nevertheless unclear whether or not the post-stroke treatment of mild hypertension is of benefit. This is because in the immediate post-stroke period, cerebral blood flow autoregulation is disordered so that rapid reductions in BP can reduce cerebral perfusion and even cause stroke extension. Recent data from the Perindopril pROtection aGainst REcurrent Stroke Study (PROGRESS) trial suggest that treatment with ACE inhibitors in patients who have had a previous (non-acute) stroke significantly reduced mortality and cardiovascular morbidity. In this study, 6105 hypertensive and nonhypertensive patients who had a stroke (haemorrhagic or ischaemic) or TIA with no major disability within the past 5 years, were either randomized to perindopril 4mg daily, with indapamide (2.5 mg daily) added at the

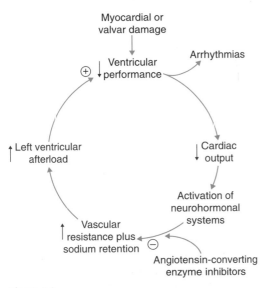

Figure 6.3
Effects of angiotensin-converting enzyme inhibitors in heart failure.

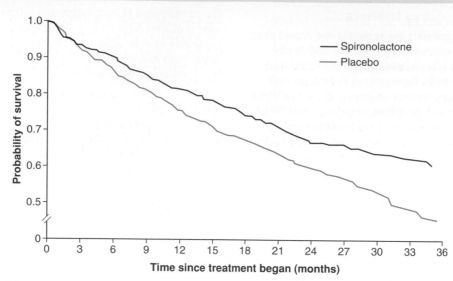

Figure 6.4
Survival curve showing a 30% reduction in all cause mortality when spironolactone was added to conventional treatment in patients with severe chronic heart failure. [Adapted from Pitt *et al*. *N Engl J Med* 1999; **341**: 709–17.]

discretion of the treating physician or matched with a placebo. After 4 years of follow-up, active treatment (60% received both drugs and 40% received perindopril alone) reduced BP by 9/4 mmHg, stroke recurrence by 28% and major cardiovascular complications by 26%, all compared to placebo. In the subgroup of active treatment patients who received both perindopril and indapamide, BP was reduced by 12/5 mmHg, and the risk of stroke was reduced by 43%. Single-drug therapy with perindopril alone reduced BP by 5/3 mmHg, but produced no significant reduction in the risk of stroke.

In cerebral infarction, low-dose aspirin (75–300 mg) should also be prescribed, although if atrial fibrillation is present warfarin should be considered.

The role of antihypertensive medication pre-, during- and post-stroke can essentially be summarized as follows:

- 'pre': many randomized controlled trials have demonstrated that it is of benefit to have hypertension treated aggressively if BP >140/85 mmHg

- 'during': it is detrimental to most to have hypertension treated aggressively. If the BP persistently exceeds 180/110 mmHg, then slow-release nifedipine 10–20 mg tablets or atenolol 25 mg should be prescribed. In patients already receiving antihypertensive medication, this is best withdrawn and only reinstated at a later stage

- 'post': this question still remains unanswered in mild hypertension even though the patients are at high risk.

The elderly

It was a widely and incorrectly held myth that a rise in BP with age was inevitable and harmless, and that isolated systolic hypertension (ISH) was actually of no consequence.

The elderly have a higher prevalence of ISH (defined as BP ≥160/<90 mmHg), occurring in >50% of people over 60 years of age. Systolic BP also rises steadily with age. These elderly hypertensive patients have a high risk of cardiovascular and cerebrovascular complications when compared to younger patients. Treatment with antihypertensive therapy reduces this risk, particularly in very high-risk groups, such as elderly non insulin-dependent diabetic hypertensives, see Figure 6.5. Treatment has been shown to reduce heart failure by 50% and possibly reduce dementia. Evidence exists that patients aged up to at least 80 years benefit from antihypertensive treatment. Newly diagnosed hypertension patients aged 80 years or more should be considered for treatment provided they are generally fit and have a reasonable life expectancy.

In the very frail elderly, assessment of the risk:benefit ratio is recommended. One ongoing trial, the Hypertension in the Very Elderly Trial (HYVET), will provide data on treating hypertension in patients aged >80 years (Figure 6.6). This is likely to be the last placebo-controlled trial and is a double blind study of over 2000 hypertensive patients aged over 80 years. The primary end point is stroke events (fatal and non fatal) and the trial is powered to determine whether there is a 35%

reduction in total stroke events between placebo and active treatment. Treatment consists of a diuretic (indapamide SR 1.5mg daily) and an additional ACE inhibitor (perindopril) if required. There is a five-year average follow up. Secondary end points to be looked at include:

- total mortality
- cardiovascular mortality
- cardiac mortality
- stroke mortality
- skeletal fracture.

> The elderly are more likely to have isolated systolic hypertension

Suggested treatment

Elderly hypertensive patients respond to non-pharmacological measures to lower BP as well as younger patients. In the elderly, low-dose diuretics and long-acting dihydropyridine

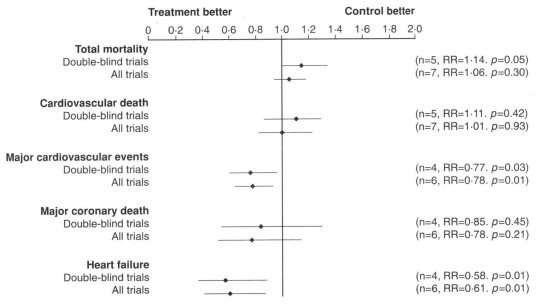

	Treatment better	Control better	

Total mortality
Double-blind trials (n=5, RR=1·14. p=0.05)
All trials (n=7, RR=1·06. p=0.30)

Cardiovascular death
Double-blind trials (n=5, RR=1·11. p=0.42)
All trials (n=7, RR=1·01. p=0.93)

Major cardiovascular events
Double-blind trials (n=4, RR=0·77. p=0.03)
All trials (n=6, RR=0·78. p=0.01)

Major coronary death
Double-blind trials (n=4, RR=0·85. p=0.45)
All trials (n=6, RR=0·78. p=0.21)

Heart failure
Double-blind trials (n=4, RR=0·58. p=0.01)
All trials (n=6, RR=0·61. p=0.01)

Figure 6.5
Antihypertensive treatment effects on cardiovascular outcomes in elderly non insulin-dependent diabetics with hypertension. [Adapted from Gueyffier et al. Lancet 1999; **353**: 793–6.]

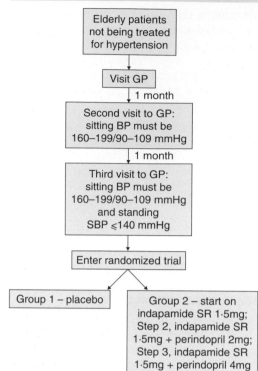

Figure 6.6
The hypertension in the very elderly trial (HYVET) protocol.

calcium antagonists are first-line drugs. Beta-blockers are less effective than thiazides as first-line treatment and meta-analyses suggest that beta-blockers decrease stroke but no other cardiovascular events in the elderly. However, the elderly have more co-morbidity and may be open to more polypharmacy and drug interactions. The concern that the elderly tolerate antihypertensive drugs poorly is probably exaggerated.

Renal disease

Renovascular disease

Renovascular disease (renal artery stenosis) is relatively uncommon, but is probably the most frequent curable cause of hypertension. ACE inhibitors may cause or worsen renal impairment in patients with critical renovascular disease. For this reason, they

should be used with caution in patients with advanced chronic renal impairment, and preferably under specialist supervision.

Clues suggesting renovascular disease include:

- onset of hypertension before the age of 30
- documented sudden onset or recent worsening of hypertension in middle age
- accelerated (malignant) hypertension
- resistant hypertension (to a three-drug regimen)
- renal impairment of unknown cause
- elevation of serum creatinine by ACE inhibitor or angiotensin II antagonist treatment
- peripheral vascular disease or severe generalized atherosclerotic disease
- recurrent pulmonary oedema or heart failure with no obvious cause.

Patients with any of these features should be referred for specialist advice because the investigations required to confirm or exclude renovascular disease are complex.

Renal failure

Many patients with renal failure have hypertension, but whether or not the hypertension is the cause of renal failure or is secondary to it often remains unclear. Hypertensive patients with elevated serum creatinine or proteinuria may have parenchymal or obstructive renal disease and should be referred for specialist evaluation. Accelerated (malignant) hypertension requires immediate hospital treatment because it causes rapid loss of renal function which can be irreversible if untreated. Otherwise, non-malignant essential hypertension does not cause renal failure. The corollary is that renal impairment, in the absence of previous accelerated phase hypertension, suggests primary renal disease or renovascular disease. In patients with chronic renal impairment, hypertension accelerates the rate of loss of renal function and good BP control is essential to retard this process.

> Patients with symptoms suggestive of renovascular disease should be referred to a specialist for complex investigations to confirm the diagnosis. This is a curable cause of hypertension

Effective treatment and renoprotection

The effective treatment of hypertension slows the progression of renal failure and it appears that ACE inhibitors are most effective in this situation. Angiotensin-converting enzyme inhibitors are both renoprotective and delay the progression of both diabetic and non-diabetic nephropathy. Whether or not ACE inhibitors have a specific renoprotective effect in non-diabetic renal failure over and above their antihypertensive action remains uncertain. Meta-analysis of all controlled trials showed a 30% reduction in the incidence of end-stage renal failure with ACE inhibitor treatment; but this may not all be explained by additional BP reduction. ACE inhibitors and angiotensin II receptor antagonists reduce proteinuria and are probably renoprotective in patients with proteinuria <3 g/day or who have rapidly progressing renal failure. These drugs may not be renoprotective in people with polycystic kidney disease.

Drugs of choice

Until we have more evidence, ACE inhibitors should be the first-choice drugs for patients with hypertensive nephropathy, except in those with bilateral renal artery stenosis (or stenosis in the artery to a single kidney). The optimal BP should be lower (BP <125/75 mmHg) for those with proteinuria >1g every 24 hours. Recent evidence suggests that the angiotensin II receptor antagonists may be a suitable alternative to ACE inhibitors, at least in diabetic nephropathy. BP is particularly salt-sensitive in patients with impaired renal function and dietary salt reduction is important. Thiazide diuretics may be ineffective in patients with renal impairment and high doses of loop diuretics (ie frusemide), are frequently required. The dose of renally excreted antihypertensive drugs may need to be adjusted.

Cardiovascular complications

The threshold for antihypertensive treatment is BP ≥140 mmHg systolic or BP ≥90 mmHg diastolic for patients with persistent proteinuria or renal impairment. Optimal BP control would be <130/85 mmHg and reducing the BP to <125/75 mmHg may produce additional benefits in patients with chronic renal disease of any aetiology and proteinuria ≥1g every 24 hours. Patients with renal failure have a very high risk of cardiovascular complications and may need aspirin or statin treatment in addition to non-pharmacological measures to reduce their cardiovascular risk burden (Figure 6.7).

Peripheral vascular disease

Hypertension is a common and important risk factor for vascular disorders, including peripheral vascular disease (PVD). Intermittent claudication is the most common symptomatic manifestation of PVD. It is also an important predictor of cardiovascular death, increasing it by three-fold and increasing all-cause mortality by two- to five-fold. About 2–5% of hypertensive patients have intermittent

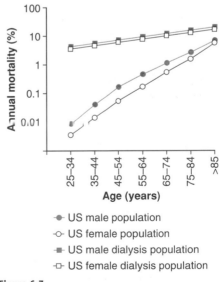

Figure 6.7
Cardiovascular mortality in dialysis patients. [Adapted from Foley *et al. Am J Kidney Dis* 1998; **32(suppl 3):** 112–19.]

claudication at presentation and this increases with age. Similarly, 35–55% of patients with PVD at presentation also have hypertension. Patients who suffer from hypertension with PVD have a greatly increased risk of MI and stroke. Apart from the epidemiological associations, hypertension also contributes to the pathogenesis of atherosclerosis – the basic pathological process underlying PVD. Peripheral vascular disease is exacerbated by:

- increases in serum lipid concentrations
- smoking.

> Hypertension is found in one-third to one-half of patients with PVD, and patients with both conditions have a much greater risk of suffering a stroke or myocardial infarction

Hypertension in common with PVD is associated with abnormalities of haemostasis and lipids, leading to an increased atherothrombotic state.

Hypertension and PVD incidence

None of the large antihypertensive treatment trials have adequately addressed whether or not a reduction in BP causes a decrease in PVD incidence. There is an obvious need for such outcome studies, especially as the two conditions are frequently encountered together but the association is often forgotten. Vasodilators, eg calcium antagonists and alpha-blockers, are useful agents in such patients. Calcium channel blockers may modestly improve the symptoms of claudication. There is the misconception that beta-blockers may worsen peripheral vascular disease, but trials comparing beta-blockers with a placebo did not significantly influence claudication distance. Nevertheless, they should probably be avoided in patients with rest pain or gangrene.

Prescribing ACE inhibitors

Angiotensin-converting enzyme inhibitors should be used with caution as there may be undiagnosed atheromatous renal artery stenosis (see above). In patients with PVD, an 'exquisite'

or over-rapid fall in BP in response to an ACE inhibitor, or a significant rise in serum creatinine levels, is a strong indicator of underlying renal artery stenosis.

> Beta-blockers should be avoided in hypertensive PVD patients with rest pain or gangrene

Ethnic groups

The ethnic differences in the incidence, pathophysiology and management of hypertension are particularly pertinent to the Afro-Caribbean population; they have a high prevalence of hypertension and associated complications such as strokes and renal impairment. The lack of large, long-term prospective randomized trials with hard outcome data has made it difficult to ascertain the precise benefits for the different antihypertensive agents in specific ethnic groups. There is also the difficulty of defining a solely Afro-Caribbean or white population, as many subgroups may exist within each ethnic group.

There are clear ethnic differences in cardiovascular disease (CVD) and its risk factors. Despite an increased prevalence of both hypertension and diabetes, the overall risk of CAD in the Afro-Caribbean male population is lower than in white males in:

- Europe
- the Caribbean
- North America (to a lesser extent).

By contrast, Indo-Asians have an excess prevalence of CAD. This contrast may be due to a multitude of reasons, although many of the traditional risk factors do not fully explain the ethnic differences in CVD and stroke.

> Ethnic differences are important in how hypertension is managed, especially in Afro-Caribbean people, and also for the risk factors associated with CVD

Afro-Caribbeans

Hypertension is known to occur more frequently in Afro-Caribbean populations and is associated with a higher incidence of cerebrovascular and renal complications. Strokes are more common and hypertension-associated end-stage renal failure is up to 20-times more frequent in Afro-Caribbean patients than non-Afro-Caribbeans.

In addition, there is a greater tendency to develop LVH; Afro-Caribbean patients with mild hypertension have a two-fold higher prevalence of LVH compared to non-Afro-Caribbeans with comparable BP levels. In the west Birmingham malignant hypertension register, there was an excess of Afro-Caribbean patients with malignant hypertension who tended to present with higher blood pressure and more severe renal impairment.

These patients had a worse overall median survival rate and an increased rate of progression to dialysis. Therefore, Afro-Caribbean patients with malignant hypertension did not do worse simply because they were Afro-Caribbean, but appeared to have poorer BP control and more complications, such as renal damage.

> Afro-Caribbean patients are 20-times more likely to develop hypertension-associated end-stage renal failure than Caucasian patients

Sodium sensitivity

Hypertensive Afro-Caribbean patients exhibit:

- enhanced sodium retention
- a higher incidence of salt-sensitive hypertension
- a higher incidence of expanded plasma volume
- a higher prevalence of low plasma renin activity.

For this reason, hypertension in Afro-Caribbeans is often sensitive to dietary salt restriction. In patients with no evidence of target organ damage, a low-salt diet may occasionally be sufficient to control BP. Reduced sodium–potassium ATPase activity, combined with a tendency towards increased intracellular sodium and calcium concentrations, is also associated with hypertension in Afro-Caribbean patients. In addition, proteinuria has been observed more frequently in African-Americans compared to white patients with similar creatinine levels. Control of dietary sodium should be combined with other non-pharmacological measures including weight control, alcohol moderation and regular exercise.

Drugs acting on the renin–angiotensin system

Afro-Caribbean patients tend to have lower levels of renin than Caucasians (Figure 6.8) and tend to respond less well to drugs that act on the renin–angiotensin system, such as beta-blockers, ACE inhibitors and angiotensin II antagonists. In contrast, they respond well to calcium antagonists, alpha-blockers and diuretics. Where there are clear indications for these agents, such as post-myocardial infarction or heart failure, they should not be denied ACE inhibitors and beta-blockers. Indeed, Afro-Caribbean patients may respond to ACE-inhibition or beta-blockade given in combination with drugs that activate the renin–angiotensin system, ie diuretics, calcium channel blockers or alpha-blockers.

South Asians

South Asians (from the Indian sub-continent) have a high prevalence of hypertension, obesity, insulin resistance and type II diabetes, giving rise to the so-called 'metabolic syndrome'. This ethnic group is at a particularly high risk of CHD. The response to antihypertensive drug treatment in South Asian patients is similar to that in white Europeans although data are limited.

One recent study (POSATIV) conducted in British Indo-Asians randomized hypertensives on background bendrofluazide therapy to valsartan or placebo. Valsartan treatment resulted in a mean BP reduction of 15.6/9.3 mmHg.

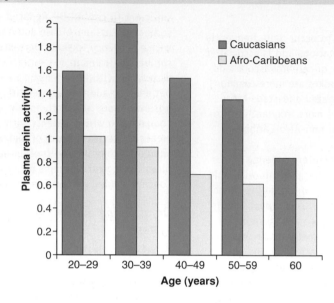

Figure 6.8
Plasma renin in Afro-Caribbean and Caucasian hypertensives.

Good control of BP is particularly important in those with diabetes and aspirin and/or statin treatment may be indicated for those at high risk of CHD.

Hyperlipidaemia

The best strategy for patients at high cardiovascular risk with hyperlipidaemia and hypertension is to treat both with different drugs, and not worry too much about small changes in cholesterol. In patients at a high risk of CVD, HMG coenzyme A inhibitors (statins) have been shown to reduce cardiovascular events. Because the beta-blockers and high-dose diuretics aggravate hyperlipidaemia, they should be avoided in people whose hyperlipidaemia is difficult to control. However, in reality, the clinical effect of these drugs on lipids is actually small.

Oral contraceptives

The combined oral contraceptives (OCs) have a small adverse effect on BP – approximately 5/3 mmHg. The increase in BP appears to be idiosyncratic and may occur many months or years after first using a combined OC. In a small proportion of women (approximately 1%) severe hypertension may be induced. As the BP response to any combined OC preparation is unpredictable, and there is a small increase in cardiovascular risk associated with OC use, BP should certainly be measured before starting OC use and then every six month thereafter. It should not be forgotten that OCs can increase the risk of venous thromboembolism.

Oral progestogen-only contraceptive pills (POP) do not increase BP. They have been recommended for use in women with a previous history of combined OC-induced hypertension, or those women with hypertension wishing to use an oral contraceptive.

If other risk factors for cardiovascular disease exist (eg smoking or migraine), other non-hormonal forms of contraception should be sought. In those women for whom other methods of contraception are unacceptable, changing to a POP with careful monitoring of BP is recommended. If BP remains elevated, antihypertensive therapy should be started.

Oral contraceptives (OCs) can affect hypertension slightly although in some cases hypertension can be severe. Progesterone-only pills do not raise BP and can be prescribed for women who have previously suffered OC-induced hypertension

Hormone replacement therapy

For many years, hormone replacement therapy (HRT) was considered to be contraindicated in postmenopausal women with hypertension. Many such women were not given HRT because of concerns that HRT may have an adverse effect on BP. This perception was mainly due to the effects of oral contraceptive drugs, especially the oestrogen component, in increasing BP. Differences exist between the formulation and doses of oestrogen preparations used in oral contraceptives in premenopausal women (where high-dose synthetic oestrogens are used) and HRT in postmenopausal women (where low 'replacement' doses of natural oestrogens are used). This is not inconsequential, as postmenopausal women represent the largest category of women at risk of hypertension. Nevertheless, there have been some uncertainties over the value of HRT in cardioprotection, and other risks, such as cancer and venous thromboembolism, should not be forgotten.

Hormone replacement therapy use is not usually associated with an increase in BP (Figure 6.9); it can be prescribed safely to hypertensive women, but careful supervision is necessary. A large, prospective, randomized, placebo-controlled study is probably needed to allay any final doubts. However, whether or not such a study would be feasible or ethical remains debatable. To study the effects of HRT on BP in 100 symptomatic hypertensive postmenopausal women, it would be necessary to screen about 1000 symptomatic postmenopausal women. In fact, more than 1000 women would need to be screened to find those that are actually symptomatic and HRT would have to be withheld in 50% of the final 100 in a placebo-controlled study.

There is no evidence at present to suggest that HRT increases blood pressure

Treating hypertension in conjunction with HRT

Hormone replacement therapy is certainly not contraindicated for women with hypertension. Women with hypertension should not be denied access to HRT as long as BP levels can be controlled by antihypertensive medication. In view of the lack of consensus in the prescribing habits of HRT, suitable guidelines are as follows:

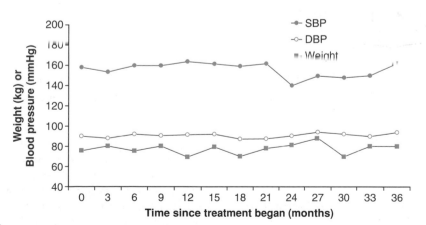

Figure 6.9
Hormone replacement therapy in hypertensive women – effects on the systolic and diastolic blood pressure. [Adapted from Lip *et al. J Hum Hypertens* 1994; **8**: 491–4.]

- All clinicians should measure BP before prescribing HRT.

- In a normotensive postmenopausal woman, BP should be measured annually following the start of HRT. One exception may be the use of premarin, where a follow-up BP measurement should probably be made at three months (in view of reports of a possible rare idiosyncratic rise in BP).

- In hypertensive menopausal women, BP should be measured initially and at least at six-monthly intervals thereafter. If BP is labile or difficult to control, three-monthly measurements should be taken. If a hypertensive woman on HRT demonstrates a rise in BP, careful monitoring or observation and perhaps an alteration or increase of their antihypertensive treatment should be considered.

Anaesthesia and surgery

The issues regarding hypertension and anaesthesia can be related to the evaluation of the BP itself (pre-operative) and the use of antihypertensive agents (intra- and post-operative). Many non-urgent surgical procedures are postponed unnecessarily when patients are erroneously diagnosed as hypertensive. In fact they are simply exhibiting anxiety-related white-coat hypertension caused by admission to hospital.

Criteria for anaesthesia use

If the patient has mild asymptomatic hypertension with no target organ damage and is otherwise fit and well, then he or she is at no particular risk in the perioperative period. In contrast, patients with severe hypertension, especially those with target organ damage, are at risk of perioperative complications (including arrhythmias or myocardial infarction). If BP >180/110 mmHg and/or LVH is present on the ECG, elective surgery should be postponed until the patient has been fully assessed and better BP control has been achieved. Parenteral control of hypertension is rarely needed because patients are usually on bed rest and receiving opioid analgesia, which reduce BP.

Suspension of antihypertensive medication

Care is needed in those patients taking particular antihypertensive drugs as some anaesthetic agents may have a hypotensive effect. The ACE inhibitors may block the response of the renin–angiotensin system, resulting in hypotension after blood loss. The beta-blockers may block the compensatory rise in heart rate associated with fluid loss. However, beta-blockers should not be stopped in the perioperative period because this class of drug has benefits in preventing post-operative arrhythmia, including atrial fibrillation. In patients with coronary artery disease, stopping the beta-blocker may provoke myocardial ischaemia. In those cases where antihypertensive drugs have to be stopped because the patient should not take them, they should be started again as soon as is practically possible.

Children

Hypertension is a rare problem in children and, where present, it is usually the result of another condition, possibly renal or vasculitic diseases (Table 6.1). Children with systemic illness should have their BP checked. It is possible that the origin of adult essential hypertension starts in childhood or even infancy.

Children whose BP exceeds the 90th percentile for their age need careful rechecking and if they exceed the 95th percentile, referral to hospital specialists and detailed investigation is mandatory.

Table 6.1
Causes of hypertension in children

Cause	Percentage
Renal parenchymal disease	75
Renal artery disease	10
Aortic coarctation	8
Endocrine causes	7

> In children, hypertension is often associated with another condition, usually renal or vasculitic disease

Measuring blood pressure

It is not considered justifiable to screen for hypertension in all children. Children with an initially high BP tend to show a faster rise with advancing age, especially when obese. Under the age of three, BP measurement can only be achieved with Doppler-flow equipment. BP should be measured with the child in a comfortable sitting position (although infants may be supine), with the right arm exposed and supported at the level of the heart. An appropriate sized cuff must be used. However, phase V sounds may be difficult to obtain in children. The guidelines therefore accept the Korotkoff sounds of K4 diastolic BP in the standards for infants and children aged from three years to 12 years, and K5 diastolic BP for adolescents aged from 13 to 18 years. The fourth and fifth Korotkoff diastolic sounds should still be recorded if both are heard.

Suggested treatment

As with general management of hypertension, non-pharmacological therapy should be initiated along with salt restriction and diet control. Beta-blockers, calcium antagonists and alpha-blockers are generally safe for children to use. However, thiazides are thought to have long-term metabolic effects and so are best avoided in children. The ACE inhibitors should be used with caution in children with renal disease.

Further reading

Adler AI, Stratton IM, Neil HA et al. Association of systolic blood pressure with macrovascular and microvascular complications of type 2 diabetes (UKPDS 36): prospective observational study. BMJ 2000; 321: 412–19.

Chung NA, Lip GYH, Beevers DG. Hypertension in old age. CPD Journal Intern Med 2001; 2: 46–9.

Cohn JN, Tognoni G. A randomized trial of the angiotensin-receptor blocker valsartan in chronic heart failure. N Engl J Med 2001; 345: 1667–75.

Cost effectiveness analysis of improved blood pressure control in hypertensive patients with type 2 diabetes: UKPDS 40. UK Prospective Diabetes Study Group. BMJ 1998; 317: 720–6.

Edmunds E, Lip GYH. Cardiovascular risk in women: the cardiologist's perspective. QJM 2000; 93: 135–45.

Efficacy of atenolol and captopril in reducing risk of macrovascular and microvascular complications in type 2 diabetes: UKPDS 39. UK Prospective Diabetes Study Group. BMJ 1998; 317: 713–20.

Felmeden DC, Lip GYH, Beevers G. Calcium antagonists in diabetic hypertension. Diabetes Obes Metab 2001; 3: 311–18.

Gibbs CR, Beevers DG, Lip GYH. The management of hypertensive disease in black patients. QJM 1999; 92: 187–92.

Intensive blood-glucose control with sulphonylureas or insulin compared with conventional treatment and risk of complications in patients with type 2 diabetes (UKPDS 33). UK Prospective Diabetes Study (UKPDS) Group. Lancet 1998; 352: 837–53.

Lip GYH, Beevers M, Beevers DG, Dillon MJ. The measurement of blood pressure and the detection of hypertension in children and adolescents. J Hum Hypertens 2001; 15: 419–23.

Patel J, Leaback R. Patients of Southern Asian descent treated with valsartan (POSATIV) study. Br J Cardiol 2002; 9: 351–4.

PROGRESS Collaborative Group. Randomised trial of a perindopril-based blood-pressure-low-ering regimen among 6,105 individuals with previous stroke or transient ischaemic attack. Lancet 2001; 358: 1033–41.

Stratton IM, Adler AI, Neil HA et al. Association of glycaemia with macrovascular and microvascular complications of type 2 diabetes (UKPDS 35): prospective observational study. BMJ 2000; 321: 405–12.

Tight blood pressure control and risk of macrovascular and microvascular complications in type 2 diabetes: UKPDS 38. UK Prospective Diabetes Study Group. BMJ 1998; 317: 703–13.

Vora JP, Ibrahim HA, Bakris GL. Responding to the challenge of diabetic nephropathy: the historic evolution of detection, prevention and management. J Hum Hypertens 2000; 14: 667–85.

Yusuf S, Sleight P, Pogue J et al. Effects of an angiotensin-converting-enzyme inhibitor, ramipril, on cardiovascular events in high-risk patients. The Heart Outcomes Prevention Evaluation Study Investigators. N Engl J Med 2000; 342: 145–53.

7. Hypertension in pregnancy

Introduction
Pre-existing essential hypertension
Secondary hypertension
Pregnancy-induced hypertension
Pre-eclampsia
Eclampsia
Choice of antihypertensive therapy
Further pregnancy

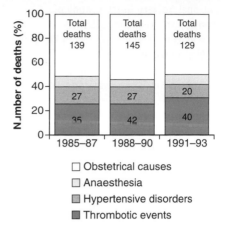

Figure 7.1
Causes of maternal deaths in the UK from 1985 to 1993.

Introduction

The management of hypertension in pregnancy
is a specialist area and a detailed treatise is
beyond the scope of this book. Hypertension
occurs in around 5% of all pregnancies.
However, this covers a wide range of
conditions that carry different implications for
pregnancy outcome and require different
management strategies. Raised blood pressure
(BP) may also be a marker of underlying
maternal disease or it may be a consequence
of pregnancy itself. It is important to
remember that hypertension in pregnancy
affects the fetus as well as the mother. It can
result in fetal growth retardation and, if
severe, both maternal and fetal morbidity and
mortality (Figure 7.1). If recognized early and
managed appropriately, many of these
complications can be reduced. Hypertension
may be the first sign of impending pre-
eclampsia – a potentially more serious
condition of the second half of pregnancy and
the puerperium. When measuring BP in
pregnant ladies, diastolic BP should be
measured at the disappearance of all sounds
(phase V) and not at muffling (phase IV) as
recommended in the past.

Consequences

Hypertensive diseases in pregnancy, including
pre-eclampsia, remain major causes of maternal
and fetal mortality in the UK (the mortality rate
is around 2%). Although maternal mortality due
to hypertension has fallen markedly over the
past three decades, eclampsia remains an
important cause of a significant number of
deaths. Eclampsia is responsible for one-sixth of
all maternal deaths and a doubling of perinatal
mortality. Despite accurate figures on the
effects of raised BP, the precise causes of
hypertension in pregnancy are unknown, and
eclampsia has been referred to as the 'disease of
theories'.

> Hypertensive diseases during pregnancy have a
> maternal and fetal mortality rate of 2%

Classification

There have been several attempts at classifying
hypertension in pregnancy, although none is
entirely satisfactory. This is partly because the
diagnoses are often made in retrospect after the
pregnancy is over. It is important to understand
the different types of hypertension in pregnancy
not least because their prognosis differs widely.
The current classification is based on the

International Society for the Study of
Hypertension in Pregnancy (ISSHP)
recommendations (Table 7.1). In 1997, Brown
and Biddle published a comparison of the
criteria of the Australasian Society for the Study
of Hypertension in Pregnancy and the
International Society for the Study of
Hypertension, studying 17,657 consecutive
pregnancies of which 1183 (6.7%) were
complicated by hypertension (Figure 7.2).

In the above classification the term 'pregnancy-
induced hypertension' is abolished. Some of
these would have chronic hypertension while
others have mild early pre-eclampsia.

Pre-existing essential hypertension

This is otherwise referred to as chronic
hypertension and is present before the 20th
week of pregnancy. It is assumed the mother had
pre-existing hypertension, although often no

Table 7.1 •
A simple classification of the hypertensive disorders of pregnancy
Raised blood pressure (>140/90 mmHg) before 20 weeks' gestation
• known chronic hypertension   – essential   – renal (glomerulonephritis, pyelonephritis, polycystic kidney disease)   – renovascular (fibromuscular dysplasia)   – adrenal (phaeochromocytoma)   • presumed chronic hypertension
Raised blood pressure (>140/90 mmHg) after 20 weeks' gestation
• chronic hypertension   • mild non-proteinuric pre-eclampsia   • proteinuric pre-eclampsia   • pre-eclampsia complicating chronic hypertension

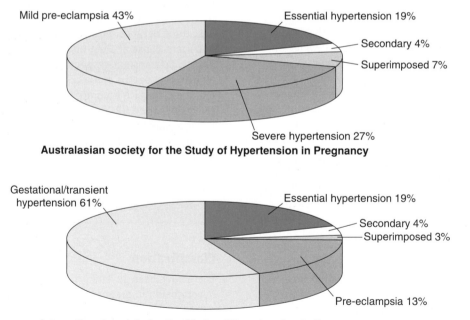

Australasian society for the Study of Hypertension in Pregnancy

(Mild pre-eclampsia 43%, Essential hypertension 19%, Secondary 4%, Superimposed 7%, Severe hypertension 27%)

International society for the Study of Hypertension in Pregnancy

(Gestational/transient hypertension 61%, Essential hypertension 19%, Secondary 4%, Superimposed 3%, Pre-eclampsia 13%)

Figure 7.2
Classifications of the hypertensive syndromes of pregnancy: the Australasian Society for the Study of Hypertension in Pregnancy classification and the International Society for the Study of Hypertension in Pregnancy classification. [Adapted from Brown *et al. J Hypertens* 1997; **15**: 1049–54.]

data are available. For this reason, chronic hypertension refers to long-term hypertension that is not confined to or caused by pregnancy, but may be revealed for the first time during pregnancy. About 5% of women of childbearing age have chronic pre-existing hypertension, which is usually mild. In women in their late 30's and 40's, this figure approaches 10%. Mild essential hypertension in pregnancy does not appear to carry a bad prognosis for the mother or fetus and its early treatment does not convincingly prevent the onset of pre-eclampsia. The condition is defined by the World Health Organization criteria as a BP >140/90 mmHg.

The usual 'cause' of chronic hypertension is essential hypertension. However, there may be other infrequent secondary causes.

> Chronic hypertension is long-term hypertension that is first discovered during the first 20 weeks of pregnancy, but is not caused by the pregnancy

Secondary hypertension

This is uncommon, but is accounted for by certain causes in younger people, such as:

- phaeochromocytoma
- renal disease
- primary hyperaldosteronism.

For example, phaeochromocytoma is well-described in association with pregnancy and is associated with a poor maternal and fetal outcome. Hypertension associated with renal disease may exacerbate renal impairment, resulting in poor outcome of the pregnancy, deterioration of renal function across pregnancy and subsequent sub-fertility.

Pregnancy-induced hypertension

Pregnancy-induced hypertension usually develops after the 20th week of pregnancy and usually resolves 10 days after delivery. For this diagnosis to be made, the BP must be documented to be normal both before and after pregnancy.

The definitions of pregnancy-induced hypertension vary. The ISSHP defines pregnancy-induced hypertension as a single diastolic (Phase V) BP >110 mmHg or two readings of >90 mmHg at least four hours apart, occurring after the 20th week of pregnancy. The US National High Blood Pressure Education Program defines it as a rise of >15 mmHg diastolic or 30 mmHg systolic compared to readings taken in early pregnancy. A concise clinical definition by Davey and MacGillivray describes the condition as 'the occurrence of a BP of 140/90 mmHg or more on at least two separate occasions a minimum of six hours apart in a woman known to have been normotensive before this time, and in whom the BP has returned to normal limits by the sixth postpartum week'.

The threshold at which drug treatment is recommended is emphatically not 140/90 mmHg. Many young pregnant women may in fact show the BP increase required for the diagnosis of pre-eclampsia without their BP increasing to 140/90 mmHg.

Pregnancy-induced hypertension affects up to 25% of women in their first pregnancy and in 10% of subsequent pregnancies.

> Pregnancy-induced hypertension can be defined as a BP of ≥140/90 mmHg measured on at least two separate occasions at least six hours apart, when the patient had been normotensive before pregnancy

If pregnancy-induced hypertension is mild and does not progress to pre-eclampsia or eclampsia, the prognosis is usually good. However, women who develop hypertension early in the second half of pregnancy are likely to progress to pre-eclampsia. They may develop proteinuria, thrombocytopenia or oedema and therefore need an early delivery.

Pre-eclampsia

Pregnancy-induced hypertension (BP >140/90 mmHg) after the 20th week of pregnancy that is associated with proteinuria (>300 mg/L), is often referred to as pre-eclampsia. This commonly occurs in primigravidas in the second half of pregnancy and marks a severe, acute change in the mother's condition. Although pre-eclampsia is defined as presenting after 20 weeks, it may often occur earlier or become evident only after delivery. The incidence of proteinuric pre-eclampsia is approximately one in 20–30 pregnancies in the UK.

> Proteinuric pre-eclampsia occurs in one in every 20–30 pregnancies in the UK

Risk factors

The risk factors for pre-eclampsia include both fetal-specific and maternal-specific factors (Table 7.2). For example, pre-eclampsia is more common in primigravidae, those aged under 20 years or over 35 years, or in women with previous severe pre-eclampsia. It is thought there is also a genetic predisposition to pre-eclampsia. Pre-eclampsia is also more common in women who are overweight and of short stature, and in women with chronic hypertension – especially those with associated chronic renal disease. Women with chronic hypertension are three to seven times more likely to develop higher BP and proteinuria (often referred to as 'superimposed pre-eclampsia') than normotensive women.

The patient is usually symptomatic with frontal headaches and visual symptoms (jagged, angular flashes at the periphery of her visual fields, loss of vision in some areas) due to cerebral oedema. There is often epigastric pain due to hepatic oedema and occasionally an itch over the mask region of the face.

> Short, overweight women and women with chronic hypertension are most susceptible to pre-eclampsia

Clinical signs

On examination, BP may be high and there is a sharp increase in proteinuria. Hypertension

Table 7.2
Pathogenesis of pre-eclampsia – failure of the normal demuscularizationof the uterine spiral arteries in early pregnancy

- Predisposing factors:
  – prior hypertension
  – prior diabetes mellitus
  – increased insulin resistance
  – increased testosterone
  – increased triglycerides, decreased HDL & increased small dense LDL
  – african origin
  – first pregnancy
  – changed paternity
  – multiple pregnancy
  – hydatidiform mole
  – fetal chromosomal abnormalities
  – placental hydrops
- Pathophysiological and clinical aspects:
  – raised blood pressure
  – proteinuria
  – reduced multi-organ perfusion
  – reduced uterine blood flow
  – increased sensitivity to pressor agents
  – vasospasm
  – reduced plasma volume
  – increased extravascular fluid volume
  – activation of coagulation cascade
  – platelet activation
  – microthrombi formation

[Adapted from Roberts and Cooper. *Lancet* 2001; **357**: 53–6]

usually precedes proteinuria but the converse is occasionally encountered.

BPs are usually unstable at rest and circadian rhythm is altered, initially with a loss of physiological nocturnal dipping; in severe cases there is 'reverse dipping' with the highest BP seen at night.

Early papilloedema may be seen on fundoscopy. There may be increased and brisk reflexes and clonus. Oedema is a less reliable diagnostic feature as mild pre-tibial and facial oedema are commonly found in normal pregnancy. Urgent antihypertensive and anticonvulsant treatment is needed. It should be noted that pregnancy-induced hypertension with or without proteinuria may be superimposed on chronic hypertension.

The presence of oedema is not a reliable diagnostic feature of pre-eclampsia as pre-tibial and facial oedema are often seen in a normal pregnancy

Eclampsia

Eclampsia is a hypertensive emergency associated with a high incidence of both maternal and fetal death. This is a convulsive condition usually associated with proteinuric pregnancy-induced hypertension and occurs in about one in 500 pregnancies.

Clinical signs

The condition resembles other forms of hypertensive encephalopathy, with similar symptoms including:

- headache
- nausea
- vomiting
- convulsions.

BP is invariably high and proteinuria >300 mg/L is almost always present. There may be gross oedema and convulsions – if they occur, they usually develop in labour or in the puerperium. Auras, epigastric pain, apprehension and hyperreflexia may precede the convulsions, with little or no warning in many cases.

After intense tonic-clonic seizures, the patient may become stuporose or comatose. Another complication common to eclampsia and hypertensive encephalopathy is cortical blindness, which results from petechial haemorrhages and focal oedema in the occipital cortex. Further complications include:

- pulmonary oedema
- renal failure
- hepatic failure
- retinal detachment
- cerebrovascular accidents.

Choice of antihypertensive therapy

Methyldopa remains the antihypertensive drug of choice for idiopathic hypertension or pre-eclampsia because of its long and extensive use without reports of serious adverse effects on the fetus. Calcium antagonists (especially nifedipine) and the vasodilator hydralazine are common second line drugs. Labetalol (alpha-blocker and beta-blocker) is also widely used as a second-line agent, particularly for resistant hypertension in the third trimester. However, angiotensin-converting enzyme (ACE) inhibitors and angiotensin II antagonists are contraindicated in pregnancy due to multiple adverse effects on the fetus. Beta-blockers, such as atenolol, may result in small babies (Figure 7.3).

Contraindicated drug therapy

Before 28 weeks gestation, beta-blockers are not widely used because of concerns that they may inhibit fetal growth. The diuretics reduce the incidence of pre-eclampsia, although no benefit was shown on fetal outcome and, in theory at least, they further reduce the already decreased circulatory blood volume in women with pre-eclampsia. ACE inhibitors and

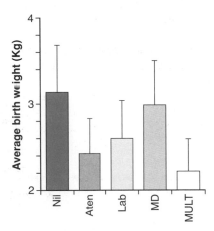

Figure 7.3
Antihypertensive drugs and fetal growth. Aten, atenolol; Lab, labetolol; MD, methyldopa; MULT, multiple drugs.
[Adapted from Lydakis *et al*. *Am J Hypertens* 1999; **12**: 541–7.]

angiotensin II receptor antagonists should be avoided because they may affect the fetus, causing:

- oligohydramnios
- renal failure
- hypotension
- intrauterine death.

Hypertensive women who are planning a pregnancy or who become pregnant while on antihypertensive treatment should be advised to change their therapy to one of the drugs recommended as safe for the treatment of hypertension in pregnancy (Table 7.3).

Use of prophylactic aspirin

The Australasian Society for the Study of Hypertension in Pregnancy (ASSHP) recommends the use of prophylactic low-dose aspirin from early pregnancy in the following groups:

- women who had prior fetal loss after the first trimester due to placental insufficiency
- women who had severe fetal growth retardation in a preceding pregnancy either due to pre-eclampsia or unexplained causes
- women who had severe early onset pre-eclampsia in a previous pregnancy requiring delivery at or before 32 weeks gestation.

Table 7.3
Drug treatments during pregnancy

- Contraindicated
  - ACE inhibitors
  - calcium channel blockers in mild hypertension
  - thiazides
  - atenolol, propranolol
- Probably safe
  - methyldopa, particularly in asthmatic mothers
  - alpha-blockers
  - some beta-blockers, eg labetalol oxprenolol, pindolol
  - nifedipine in severe cases
- Emergency
  - intravenous and intramuscular drugs, eg hydralazine, labetalol
  - anticonvulsants
  - magnesium sulphate

Aspirin is not indicated routinely for healthy nulliparous women, women with mild chronic hypertension and women with established pre-eclampsia.

Pre-eclampsia

Urgent transfer to a specialized maternity unit with an adequate special care baby unit is indicated together with antihypertensive and anticonvulsant therapy. Diazepam and magnesium sulphate prevent fits and reduce BP.

Eclampsia

The first line of management is to control the seizures. If at home, the woman should be laid on her side and an airway established. Intravenous diazepam, usually 20–40 mg, is used. Occasionally phenytoin is used to prevent recurrence of fits. In the US, magnesium sulphate is a popular choice as an anticonvulsant in eclampsia, and its use has now been advocated as the optimal first-line drug. Intravenous hydralazine is a useful antihypertensive drug of first choice, given as a 5 mg bolus at 20 minutes or as an infusion of 25 mg in 500 ml of Hartmann's solution. The dose is titrated against the woman's BP. An alternative is an intravenous infusion of labetalol. If the woman is in labour or induction is considered, an epidural anaesthetic may be helpful to both lower the BP and reduce the tendency to fit by reducing the pain of uterine contractions. The ultimate treatment of eclampsia is urgent delivery of the baby.

> Magnesium sulphate is the first-line drug to treat eclampsia seizures

Further pregnancy

Mothers who have had pre-eclampsia during a first pregnancy should be warned of a 7.5% risk that it might return for their second pregnancy. A history of spontaneous or induced first trimester abortion in a first pregnancy does not confer the same relative immunity to severe pre-eclampsia in the subsequent pregnancy. Other causes of hypertension should be considered when a patient develops hypertension in pregnancy, especially if there are any unusual features or the hypertension is severe.

Women with previous pre-eclampsia who become pregnant again should be targeted for management in a joint antenatal and BP clinic. Such women are also usually regarded as being more likely to develop essential hypertension in later life and regular screening for hypertension is recommended (Table 7.4). If a woman with a history of hypertension in pregnancy wishes to use oral contraception (this is not a contraindication), careful BP monitoring is essential. The developmental status of children born to women with pre-eclampsia is usually good.

> Women who develop pre-eclampsia during their first pregnancy have a 7.5% risk of it returning for their next pregnancy, and should be monitored at joint antenatal and BP clinics

The benefits of treating hypertension in pregnancy are best summed up in Table 7.5. Clearly the best data are for the treatment of pre-eclampsia and eclampsia, with benefits for both the mother and baby, especially in the presence of severe hypertension. These uncertainties over the benefits of treatment are compounded by a recent metaanalysis suggesting that over-aggressive BP reduction in pregnancy is associated with a greater odds ratio for small for gestational-age babies and lower birth weight babies.

In a paper by von Dadelszen et al, the relationship between fetoplacental growth and the use of oral antihypertensive medication to treat mild-to-moderate pregnancy hypertension was assessed using a metaregression analysis of published data from randomized controlled trials. The change in (group) mean arterial pressure (MAP) from enrolment to delivery was compared with indicators of fetoplacental growth. They found that greater mean difference in MAP with antihypertensive therapy was associated with the birth of a higher proportion of small-for-gestational-age infants. No relation with mean placental weight was seen. This analysis therefore suggests that treatment-induced falls in maternal BP may adversely affect fetal growth. In view of the small maternal benefits that are likely to be derived from therapy, more information on the relative maternal and fetal benefits and risks of oral antihypertensive drug treatment of mild-to-moderate pregnancy hypertension is required.

Table 7.4
Laboratory tests used to diagnose hypertension in pregnancy

Test	Rationale
Full blood count	Haemoconcentration is found in pre-eclampsia and is an indicator of severity Decreased platelet count suggests severe pre-eclampsia
Blood film	Signs of microangiopathic haemolytic anaemia favour the diagnosis of pre-eclampsia
Urinalysis	If dipstick proteinuria of +1 or more, a quantitative measurement of 24-hour protein excretion is required Hypertensive pregnant women with proteinuria should be considered to have pre-eclampsia until proven otherwise
Biochemistry, including serum creatinine, urate and liver function tests	Abnormal or rising levels suggest pre-eclampsia and are an indicator of disease severity
Lactate dehydrogenase	Elevated levels are associated with haemolysis and hepatic involvement, suggesting severe pre-eclampsia
Serum albumin	Levels may be decreased even with mild proteinuria, perhaps due to capillary leak or hepatic involvement in pre-eclampsia

[Adapted from recommendations of the National High Blood Pressure Education Program Working Group Report on High Blood Pressure in Pregnancy. *Am J Obstet Gynecol* 1990; **163**: 1689–1712.]

Table 7.5(a)

Are there benefits of treating hypertension during pregnancy?

	Mother	Fetus
Pre-existing hypertension	Yes*	No
Pregnancy-induced hypertension	No	No
Pre-eclampsia	Yes*	Yes*

*Depending on severity

Table 7.5(b)

Antihypertensive therapy for chronic hypertension during pregnancy

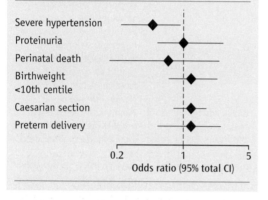

Further reading

Broughton Pipkin F, Roberts JM. Hypertension in pregnancy. *J Hum Hypertens* 2000; **14**: 705–24.

Brown MA, Buddle ML. What's in a name? Problems with the classification of hypertension in pregnancy. *J Hypertens* 1997; **15**: 1049–54.

Chung NA, Beevers DG, Lip GYH. Management of hypertension in pregnancy. *Am J Cardiovasc Drugs* 2001; **1**: 253–62.

Dekker G, Sibai B. Primary, secondary, and tertiary prevention of pre-eclampsia. *Lancet* 2001; **357**: 209–15.

Department of Health and Social Security. Report on confidential enquiries into maternal deaths in England and Wales 1982–84. London, HMSO 1986: 10–19.

Ferrer RL, Sibai BM, Mulrow CD *et al*. Management of mild chronic hypertension during pregnancy: a review. *Obstet Gynecol* 2000; **96**: 849–60.

Granger JP, Alexander BT, Bennett WA, Khalil RA. Pathophysiology of pregnancy-induced hypertension. *Am J Hypertens* 2001; **14**: 178S–185S.

Lydakis C, Lip GYH, Beevers M, Beevers DG. Atenolol and fetal growth in pregnancies complicated by hypertension. *Am J Hypertens* 1999; **12**: 541–7.

Sibai BM. Antihypertensive drugs during pregnancy. *Semin Perinatol* 2001; **25**: 159–64.

von Dadelszen P, Ornstein MP, Bull SB *et al*. Fall in mean arterial pressure and fetal growth restriction in pregnancy hypertension: a meta-analysis. *Lancet* 2000; **355**: 87–92.

8. Urgencies and emergencies

Epidemiology
Pathophysiology
Clinical features
Physical signs
Early management
Summary

Urgency - day/week
emergency - minute

Table 8.1
Hypertensive crises

- Hypertensive emergencies
  hypertensive encephalopathy
  - hypertensive left ventricular failure
  - hypertension with myocardial infarction or unstable angina
  - hypertension with aortic dissection
  - severe hypertension with subarachnoid haemorrhage or stroke
  - phaeochromocytoma crisis
  - recreational drugs (amphetamines, LSD, cocaine, ecstasy)
  - perioperative hypertension
  - severe pre-eclampsia or eclampsia
- Hypertensive urgencies
  - malignant hypertension
  - chronic renal failure
  - pre-eclampsia
  - severe non-malignant hypertension

'Hypertensive crises' are severe elevations in blood pressure (BP) and can be classified as either 'urgencies' or 'emergencies'. In hypertensive urgencies there is no evidence of acute target organ damage, while in hypertensive emergencies there is an immediate threat to the cardiovascular system and to the patient (Table 8.1). For example, malignant hypertension is associated with potentially irreversible target organ damage that occurs over days or weeks, rather than minutes, and is classified as an hypertensive urgency. Conditions that are associated with a more immediate threat to life and are considered to be true hypertensive emergencies include:

- hypertensive encephalopathy ✓
- hypertensive left ventricular failure ✓
- acute aortic dissection. ✓

It is important to have coherent strategies for the diagnosis, investigation and management of hypertensive crises, as the mortality in these patients is high and rapid treatment of hypertension may itself be hazardous. These risks are greatly increased when patients are treated with inappropriate pharmacological agents in the absence of appropriate monitoring.

Epidemiology

There has been a decline in the prevalence of hypertensive crises over the past 20 years. This is likely to be a result of more effective diagnosis and treatment of milder grades of hypertension. Malignant hypertension is now reported to be rare in western developed populations, although it is still reported to be common in some developing countries. Nevertheless, in Birmingham, UK, the incidence of malignant hypertension does not appear to have fallen substantially over the past 25 years, with an estimated annual incidence of 1 to 2 per 100,000 population (Figure 8.1).

Malignant hypertension

Hypertensive crises may present at any age, including the elderly, and recurrent clinical presentations of malignant-phase hypertension might occur. Malignant hypertension in young women has been related to both the use of the oral contraceptive pill and a history of hypertension in pregnancy. Several studies have also reported an association between cigarette smoking and malignant hypertension.

Demographic and socio-economic factors appear to be important and may contribute to the lack

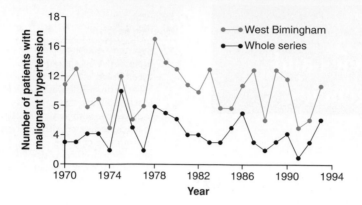

Figure 8.1
Failure of malignant hypertension to decline in Birmingham, UK.

of falling rates of malignant hypertension cases in some areas of the world. Malignant hypertension is reported to occur more frequently in patients from lower socio-economic groups and in subjects with high self-perceived 'stress' levels. Ethnicity may be important and closer examination of the Birmingham cohort reveals a high prevalence in first-generation migrant groups, including Afro-Caribbeans (mainly from Jamaica) and Asians (mainly from Punjabi-speaking areas of India and Pakistan). In this respect, the Birmingham cohort resembles other series of malignant hypertensive patients from less developed countries (eg South Africa).

A further reason for the failure of malignant hypertension to decline might be the presence of patients who have limited understanding of the nature and complications of the disease, and the importance of compliance with antihypertensive treatment.

> Hypertensive crises may be found in any age group, including the elderly, and studies have linked them to demographic and ethnic factors

Causes

Hypertensive crises are more likely to be associated with an underlying cause (see Table 8.2). Conn's syndrome (primary hyperaldosteronism) is reported to be rare in cases of malignant hypertension.

Prognosis

In the modern era, the more effective management of hypertension has lead to an improvement in five-year survival rates in developed countries – from 60–75% (Figure 8.2). Nevertheless, in developing countries, such as Nigeria, the prognosis continues to be poor with only 40% of patients surviving longer than one year.

Table 8.2
Underlying causes in studies of patients with malignant hypertension

	Glasgow	Leicester	Johannesburg	Birmingham
Follow-up year	1968–83	1974–83	1979–80	1970–93
Number of patients	139	100	62	242
Underlying causes (%)				
Essential	60	68	82	56
Renal	18	19	5	28
Renovascular	14	6	3	2
Other	8	7	10	14

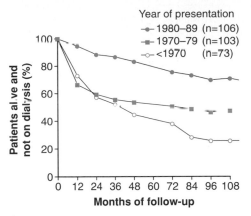

Figure 8.2
Survival of malignant hypertension. [Adapted from Lip *et al.*
J Hypertens 1995; **13**: 915.]

Early recognition

Early recognition of malignant hypertension is important as patients tend to develop overt clinical symptoms at a late stage of the disease. In the long-term, the most common causes of death in patients with a history of malignant hypertension are:

- chronic renal failure (40%)
- cerebrovascular disease (24%)
- myocardial infarction (11%)
- heart failure (10%).

Cigarette smoking exerts an adverse effect on the prognosis in patients who continue to smoke following their initial presentation. Renal function continues to deteriorate in some patients with malignant hypertension despite good BP control during follow-up. Nevertheless, the quality of the BP control does predict the long-term prognosis and BP control should be optimal, with the target being 140/80 mmHg.

> The most common causes of death in patients with a history of malignant hypertension are chronic renal failure, cerebrovascular disease, myocardial infarction and heart failure

Pathophysiology
Histology

Malignant hypertension is characterized by fibrinoid necrosis of arterioles in many sites, including:

- kidneys
- eyes
- brain
- heart
- gut.

However, this histological feature is not pathognomonic of malignant hypertension. Subintimal cellular proliferation of the interlobular arteries of the kidney is also commonly seen and this may well be important as intimal thickening may lead to luminal occlusion in these small vessels. The occlusion of these small arteries contributes to chronic renal ischaemia, leading to the renal failure that is often seen in malignant hypertension.

Microscopic examination of the arterioles reveals alternating bands of constriction and dilatation. These dilated segments are thought to represent focal areas of disruption of the vessel wall related to the rapid rise in intraluminal pressure, and these areas have been shown to be abnormally permeable to plasma proteins.

Such disruption of the vessel wall leads to the deposition of fibrin, and therefore fibrinoid necrosis. This process may lead to the further deposition of fibrin in the vessel wall and microcirculation, as well as platelet aggregation, release of growth factors and subintimal cellular proliferation. The coagulation system may also be activated, which may result in microangiopathic haemolytic anaemia – a recognized feature in some of these patients. In addition, ischaemia of the juxtaglomerular apparatus leads to activation of the renin–angiotensin system with further vasoconstriction and arteriolar damage.

> Malignant hypertension is marked by fibrinoid necrosis of arterioles in sites such as the kidneys, eyes, brain, heart and gut

> The most common symptoms of malignant hypertension are headaches and visual disturbances, with non-specific symptoms including anorexia, nausea, vomiting and abdominal pain

Cerebral autoregulation

Cerebral autoregulation is impaired in chronic hypertension and cerebrovascular disease, both common features in patients with hypertensive crises. Cerebral autoregulation is also impaired at extremely high BP levels and in hypertensive encephalopathy, probably as a result of disruption to the blood–brain barrier. This malfunction can lead to cerebral oedema. Clearly, these abnormalities of cerebral autoregulation have important implications for the practical management of hypertensive emergencies.

Clinical features and symptoms

Severe hypertension may be an incidental finding in an asymptomatic patient, although associated symptoms may be present. The presenting symptoms of malignant hypertension are variable, although headaches and visual disturbances are the most common. Initial symptoms are often non-specific and include anorexia, nausea, vomiting and abdominal pain. Breathlessness due to left ventricular failure might be present but ischaemic chest pain is less common. Aortic dissection must be considered in any patient who presents with raised BP and severe pain in the back, chest or abdomen.

Hypertensive encephalopathy is rare and usually occurs in patients with a history of hypertension that has been inadequately treated, or where previous treatment has been discontinued. It may be associated with severe headache, nausea, vomiting, visual disturbances and confusion. However, with the advent of high-resolution computed tomography scanning, it has become clear that many patients who are thought to have hypertensive encephalopathy have actually suffered an acute stroke.

Physical Signs

Retinopathy

Malignant hypertension is confirmed by the presence of advanced retinal hypertensive changes. Clinical decisions in patients with severe hypertension should be based on the presence or absence of retinopathy together with the height of the BP. The Keith, Wagener, Barker classification (see Table 3.6), originally proposed in 1939, remains the most commonly used grading system for hypertensive retinopathy. The strength of this classification was the correlation between the clinical signs and prognosis, although this grading system has a number of limitations. In particular, there is no significant difference in the long-term prognosis between grades III and IV hypertensive retinopathy.

The restrictions of this traditional classification for hypertensive retinopathy has lead to the development of a simplified grading system, which is more applicable to modern clinical practice (Table 8.3). In this grading system:

* Grade I = arteriolar narrowing and focal constriction, features which correlate with BP levels, age and general cardiovascular status.
* Grade II = the presence of retinal haemorrhages or exudates, cotton wool spots (with or without papilloedema). Grade II is the prognostically more significant grade (Figure 8.3).

An additional subgroup of patients has been identified who have isolated bilateral papilloedema in association with severe hypertension (Figure 8.4). The clinical characteristics of these patients are similar to those with 'conventional' malignant

Table 8.3
Revised grading system for hypertensive retinopathy

	Retinal changes	Hypertensive category	Prognosis
Grade I 'Non-malignant'	Generalized arteriolar narrowing Focal constriction (NB *not* arterio-venous nipping)	Established hypertension	May depend on height of blood pressure, but age and other concomitant cardiovascular risk factors are equally important
Grade II 'Malignant'	Haemorrhages, hard exudates, cotton wool spots ± optic disc swelling	Accelerated or malignant hypertension with retino-vascular damage present*	Most cases die within 2 years if untreated In treated patients, median survival rate is now >12 years

*To fulfil the criteria of Grade II, retino-vascular damage should be present in both eyes. Note that if carotid occlusive disease is present, ocular blood flow may be reduced and if asymmetrical this may be sufficient to mask papilloedema or other hypertensive changes in the ipsilateral eye.

[Adapted from Dodson PM *et al.* Hypertensive retinopathy: a review of existing classification systems and a suggestion for a simplified grading system. *J Human Hypertens* 1996, **10**: 93–98.]

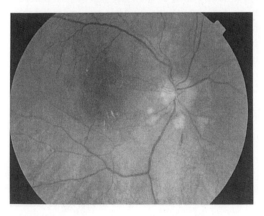 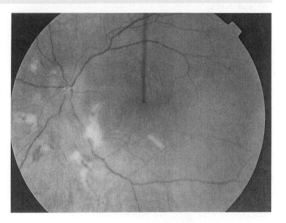

Figure 8.3
Malignant phase hypertension – retinal flame-shaped haemorrhages, cotton wool spots, exudates and papilloedema are visible.

hypertension, although they have been reported to have a shorter median survival. However, care is needed to differentiate such patients from those with benign intracranial hypertension, who are typically young, overweight and female. A computed tomography scan and lumbar puncture may be needed to ascertain the diagnosis.

Other clinical signs

In addition to the retinopathy there may be signs of left heart failure, left ventricular hypertrophy and sometimes anaemia due to associated renal failure. Asymmetrical BP

readings, absent pulses, aortic incompetence and neurological signs should raise the suspicion of acute aortic dissection. Fluctuating neurological signs, disorientation, reduced level of consciousness, neurological deficit and focal or generalized seizures are all potential manifestations of hypertensive encephalopathy.

Early management
Malignant hypertension

A gradual reduction in BP is important as the brain, kidneys and heart have protective vascular

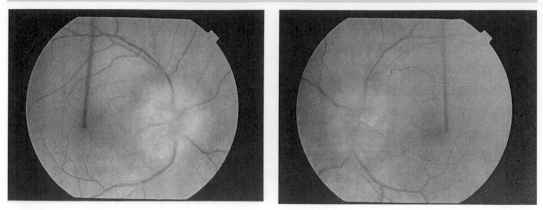

Figure 8.4
Lone papilloedema in a patient with severe hypertension, showing bilateral optic disc swelling and no other significant retinal features.

autoregulatory mechanisms, which maintain a constant blood flow to the organs. Consequently, over-rapid BP reductions are potentially hazardous and may lead to cerebral, renal or myocardial infarction (MI), while visual loss is also a recognized complication of over-rapid treatment.

In the absence of acute life-threatening target organ damage, immediate BP reduction with parenteral drugs is not indicated. Indeed, this form of treatment may place the patient at unnecessary risk, as serious and sometimes fatal complications of treatment have been reported with almost all anti-hypertensive drugs.

Parenteral therapy

Parenteral therapy requires high-dependency monitoring and should be restricted to severe emergencies where complications such as hypertensive encephalopathy, left ventricular failure and aortic dissection are present. In most cases of malignant hypertension the patient should be admitted to hospital and the BP lowered gradually over the first few days with oral therapy only.

First-line drugs

An appropriate first-line oral agent is slow-release nifedipine (10–20 mg in tablet form), which is a simple, effective and safe treatment and which does not significantly alter cerebral blood flow.

Nifedipine capsules and sublingual nifedipine must not be used as their use has been reported to be associated with dramatic and unpredictable falls in BP, leading to cerebral and myocardial ischaemia. Intensive care monitoring is not usually necessary. The dose of slow-release nifedipine may be repeated or increased at intervals of 6–12 hours, aiming for a gradual reduction in BP of 20–25% in the first 24 hours. The aim is a diastolic BP of around 100 mmHg over the next few days.

> Slow-release nifedipine in tablet form is a first-line drug for malignant hypertension that does not alter cerebral blood flow significantly, however, sublingual capsules must not be used

Combination treatment

Combination treatment is usually required in the long term. In the absence of contraindications, beta-blockers (eg atenolol) are an appropriate additional antihypertensive agent. It is sensible to start with small doses, such as atenolol 25 mg daily, increasing as necessary. The combination of atenolol and nifedipine is often a well-tolerated and effective regime.

Angiotensin-converting enzyme inhibitors

Angiotensin-converting enzyme (ACE) inhibitors may produce rapid and dangerous falls in BP (particularly in patients with renovascular disease which might not be diagnosed in the acute situation) and are not recommended as first-line treatment. Diuretics should be restricted to those with evidence of fluid-overload as patients with malignant hypertension are often volume depleted secondary to pressure-related diuresis and activation of the renin–angiotensin system. In severe renal failure, haemodialysis or peritoneal dialysis may be indicated, particularly where there is gross fluid retention.

Hypertensive encephalopathy

Sodium nitroprusside

Sodium nitroprusside is the drug of choice when neurological damage is thought to be imminent. It is a potentially dangerous drug and should only be administered in a high dependency unit with cardiac and BP monitoring. Nitroprusside is administered as a continuous titrated infusion, which is increased to achieve a diastolic BP of 90–110 mmHg over two to three hours. Thiocyanate is the toxic metabolite of nitroprusside and its accumulation is more rapid in patients with renal failure.

Labetalol

Parenteral labetalol has been successfully used in the treatment of hypertensive encephalopathy, although it has been reported to cause severe and unpredictable hypotension in some patients. Intravenous nitrates are of limited value in hypertensive encephalopathy because they cause headache at the doses required to bring about a substantial reduction in BP.

Arterial vasodilators

Diazoxide and hydralazine, both arterial vasodilators, were previously popular in the management of hypertensive crises. Diazoxide, administered by rapid bolus injection, has lead to a number of cases of cerebral infarction and death, and it is now a rarely used treatment. Reflex tachycardia is associated with both diazoxide and hydralazine and these agents should be avoided in patients with known or suspected coronary disease. In all cases of suspected hypertensive encephalopathy, if a reduction in BP is not accompanied by clinical improvement, the diagnosis should be reconsidered.

Left ventricular failure

Severe increases in systemic vascular resistance may result in left ventricular failure. In addition to the conventional management with opiates or opioids and loop diuretics, sodium nitroprusside is used to reduce preload and afterload. Nitrates may also be used, but are less potent.

Unstable angina or myocardial infarction

In patients with severe hypertension and angina, intravenous nitrates are valuable as they reduce systemic vascular resistance and improve coronary perfusion. Beta-blockers administered by slow intravenous injection (for example 5 mg metoprolol repeated at intervals of 20 minutes) may be valuable when the BP is moderately raised. In severe hypertension an intravenous infusion (eg labetalol or esmolol) may be necessary. Sodium nitroprusside should be reserved for resistant cases as it may exacerbate coronary ischaemia.

Aortic dissection

The treatment of choice in type B aortic dissection (distal to the subclavian artery) is prompt and effective BP control. The aim of therapy should be to reduce the systolic BP to 100 mmHg in order to reduce aortic shear stress and limit the size of the dissection. Labetalol is an effective agent as is sodium nitroprusside in combination with a beta-blocker.

Labetalol is the main agent used to treat type B aortic dissection in hypertensive patients; sodium nitroprusside in combination with a beta-blocker is also useful.

Stroke and subarachnoid haemorrhage

Cerebral autoregulation is commonly disturbed following an acute stroke. Excessive antihypertensive treatment may only serve to worsen the cerebral damage that results from an intracerebral infarction or haemorrhage. Antihypertensive treatment may lead to rapid and dangerous falls in BP, and should only be administered for severe elevations in BP (diastolic BP >130 mmHg). In these cases, oral therapy with small doses of slow-release nifedipine or atenolol may be indicated, although parenteral treatment is almost always contraindicated.

The calcium antagonist nimodipine has beneficial effects on cerebral vasospasm following subarachnoid haemorrhage, but these effects are not related to the small fall in blood pressure.

Phaeochromocytoma

This condition is a rare cause of acute severe hypertension. The treatment of choice is the orally active, short-acting alpha-blocker prazosin or phentolamine (which may also be given by bolus injection or infusion). It is possible to subsequently add a beta-blocker to control heart rate. Labetalol has also been used, but nitroprusside should be reserved for resistant cases. Alpha-blockade is mandatory in the preoperative management of patients with phaeochromocytoma. It is used to overcome the intense vasoconstriction caused by the high circulating levels of adrenaline and noradrenaline.

Recreational drugs

The sympathomimetic drugs that can produce severe acute hypertension include:

- cocaine
- ecstasy
- amphetamines
- LSD.

Labetalol is normally effective in lowering the BP after taking these drugs, although nitroprusside and phentolamine may also be used.

Summary

Although hypertensive crises are less common in modern-day medical practice, they are associated with significant morbidity and mortality rates. This is because malignant hypertension remains a disease with a poor long-term prognosis.

In the majority of cases, rapid-onset orally active drugs are sufficient to control the BP (Table 8.4). Preparations of labetalol or sodium

Table 8.4
Drug treatment in hypertensive crises

Drug	Route	Dose	Principal indications
Nifedipine	oral	Start at 10 mg and repeat after 4–6 hours	Malignant hypertension
	oral	Maintenance 10–40 mg bid	
Atenolol	IV	Start at 25 mg Maximum 100 mg daily	Malignant hypertension
Sodium nitroprusside	IV	0.3–8 mg/kg/min Monitor levels in prolonged use	Hypertensive encephalopathy, left ventricular failure, dissecting aneurysm
Labetalol	IV	2 mg/min	Hypertensive encephalopathy, dissecting aneurysm, unstable angina or MI
Nitrates	IV	GTN 10–200 mg/min	Left ventricular failure, unstable angina with malignant hypertension

GTN, glyceryl trinitrate; MI, myocardial infarction; IV, intravenous nitroprusside are occasionally necessary in cases of resistant hypertension and true hypertensive crises. However, clinicians should be aware of the hazards associated with the over-rapid reduction of BP in these patients as well as the complications of hypertension in the first place.

Further reading

Lim KG, Isles CG, Hodsman GP *et al*. Malignant hypertension in women of childbearing age and its relation to the contraceptive pill. *Br Med J (Clin Res Ed)* 1987; **294**: 1057–9.

Lip GYH, Beevers M, Beevers DG. Complications and survival of 315 patients with malignant-phase hypertension. *J Hypertens* 1995; **13**: 915–24.

Lip GYH, Beevers M, Beevers DG. Malignant hypertension in young women is related to previous hypertension in pregnancy, not oral contraception. *QJM* 1997; **90**: 571–5.

Lip GYH, Beevers M, Beevers DG. The failure of malignant hypertension to decline: a survey of 24 years' experience in a multiracial population in England. *J Hypertens* 1994; **12**: 1297–305.

Index